Exam Preparatory Manual
Microbiology
(VIRAT)

Exam Preparatory Manual
Microbiology
(VIRAT)

Second Edition

Thanveer P MBBS
Ramki M MBBS
Vivek VK MBBS

Interns
Kerala University of Health Sciences
Government Medical College
Thrissur, Kerala, India

JAYPEE *The Health Sciences Publisher*
New Delhi | London | Panama | Philadelphia

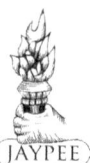

Jaypee Brothers Medical Publishers (P) Ltd

Headquarters
Jaypee Brothers Medical Publishers (P) Ltd.
4838/24, Ansari Road, Daryaganj
New Delhi 110 002, India
Phone: +91-11-43574357
Fax: +91-11-43574314
Email: jaypee@jaypeebrothers.com

Overseas Offices

J.P. Medical Ltd.
83, Victoria Street, London
SW1H 0HW (UK)
Phone: +44-20 3170 8910
Fax: +44-(0)20 3008 6180
Email: info@jpmedpub.com

JP Medical Inc.
325 Chestnut Street, Ste 412
Philadelphia, PA 19106
Phone: +1 267-519-9789
Email: support@jpmedus.com

Jaypee-Highlights Medical Publishers Inc.
City of Knowledge, Bld. 237, Clayton
Panama City, Panama
Phone: +1 507-301-0496
Fax: +1 507-301-0499
Email: cservice@jphmedical.com

Jaypee Brothers Medical Publishers (P) Ltd.
17/1-B, Babar Road, Block-B, Shaymali
Mohammadpur, Dhaka-1207, Bangladesh
Mobile: +08801912003485
Email: jaypeedhaka@gmail.com

Jaypee Brothers Medical Publishers (P) Ltd.
Bhotahity, Kathmandu, Nepal
Phone: +977-9741283608
Email: kathmandu@jaypeebrothers.com

Website: www.jaypeebrothers.com
Website: www.jaypeedigital.com

© 2016, Jaypee Brothers Medical Publishers

The views and opinions expressed in this book are solely those of the original contributor(s)/author(s) and do not necessarily represent those of editor(s) of the book.

All rights reserved. No part of this publication may be reproduced, stored or transmitted in any form or by any means, electronic, mechanical, photocopying, recording or otherwise, without the prior permission in writing of the publishers.

All brand names and product names used in this book are trade names, service marks, trademarks or registered trademarks of their respective owners. The publisher is not associated with any product or vendor mentioned in this book.

Medical knowledge and practice change constantly. This book is designed to provide accurate, authoritative information about the subject matter in question. However, readers are advised to check the most current information available on procedures included and check information from the manufacturer of each product to be administered, to verify the recommended dose, formula, method and duration of administration, adverse effects and contraindications. It is the responsibility of the practitioner to take all appropriate safety precautions. Neither the publisher nor the author(s)/editor(s) assume any liability for any injury and/or damage to persons or property arising from or related to use of material in this book.

This book is sold on the understanding that the publisher is not engaged in providing professional medical services. If such advice or services are required, the services of a competent medical professional should be sought.

Every effort has been made where necessary to contact holders of copyright to obtain permission to reproduce copyright material. If any have been inadvertently overlooked, the publisher will be pleased to make the necessary arrangements at the first opportunity.

Inquiries for bulk sales may be solicited at: jaypee@jaypeebrothers.com

Exam Preparatory Manual Microbiology (VIRAT)

First Edition: **2014**
(Published by Author)
Second Edition: **2016**

ISBN: 978-93-85891-77-9

Dedicated to

The God Almighty
Parents and Teachers

Preface to the Second Edition

As we present the second edition, we are full of emotions due to overwhelming support from our readers and teachers. VIRAT's Synopsis of Microbiology has helped the undergraduates since the last three years for the preparation of examinations in microbiology.

The second edition of 'VIRAT's Synopsis of Microbiology' has been renamed as 'Exam Preparatory Manual Microbiology (VIRAT)'. The book continues to focus on the undergraduate medical students. While we ensure that the 'must know' contents are thoroughly covered, we provide an optimum glimpse of the 'should know' curriculum for our readers. We have been careful in ensuring that the size of the book enables it to be easily readable and handy enough to be taken to the classrooms.

A number of changes have been incorporated in this edition. We welcome Dr Anand of 33rd batch and Dr Aswin Krishnamoorthy of 32nd batch, who joined us as editors.

We are grateful to our families for their support and understanding. And, finally, we thank our mentors, our juniors and readers for being the mission and the driving force for this work.

Thanveer P
Ramki M
Vivek VK

Preface to the First Edition

VIRAT's Synopsis of Microbiology is intended to help the undergraduate students. Readers can avail precise information about the important topics that are to be dealt in the MBBS curriculum. This book is based on Ananthanarayan and Paniker's Textbook of Microbiology, 9th edition, and Paniker's Textbook of Medical Parasitology, 7th edition.

Turning the pages you can see the topics are compiled under headings and subheadings, which the students find easier to understand and recall when needed. We have included tables, flowcharts and appropriate pictures along with concise notes prepared under scrutiny of experts in microbiology. We do not claim any perfection but remind you that this book mainly serves the purpose of good revision. The information is updated to the latest and if any shortcomings or errors are found, kindly give us suggestions as to how to improve the book by mailing us at virat2k14@yahoo.com.

Thanveer P
Ramki M
Vivek VK

Acknowledgments

Firstly, acknowledgment to the supreme power and our parents for guiding the intellect along the correct path.

We would also like to acknowledge the encouragement and guidance of our teachers of the Department of Microbiology.

No words can describe the immense contribution of our friends and classmates of 31st Laennec's (2011 batch), especially Ashbina K, Vinayak V, Sarath H, Sreejith Sreekumar, Nishna N, Vysakh C, Shajirmon M, Muhammed Afsal and Anoop Titus, without whose support this book would not have seen the light of the day.

We want to extend our special thanks to our juniors Aswin Krishnamoorthy, Vaisakh (32nd Hunters), Aswanth, Anand, Prasad of 33rd Flemings batch and Rahul Raveendran of 35th Khoranas batch.

At last, we wish to say that without the financial support of our college union AAGNEYA 2014–15, this book would just have remained in the form of notes.

We dedicate this book to all TMCians.

From the Publisher's Desk
We request all the readers to provide us their
valuable suggestions/errors (if any)
at: ***jppgmee@gmail.com***
so as to help us in further improvement of this book in the subsequent edition(s)

Contents

1. General Microbiology — 1
2. Sterilization and Disinfection — 4
3. Culture Media and Methods — 8
4. Bacterial Genetics — 12
5. Infection — 16
6. Immunology — 18
7. Streptococcus — 34
8. Staphylococcus — 38
9. Neisseria — 41
10. Vibrio Cholera — 45
11. Bacillus — 47
12. Clostridium — 50
13. Tetanus — 53
14. Enterobacteriaceae — 55
15. Non-sporing Anaerobes — 65
16. Bordetella Pertussis — 66
17. Haemophilus Influenzae — 68
18. Corynebacterium Diphtheria — 70
19. Pseudomonas — 72
20. Brucella — 74
21. Mycobacterium Nonmycobacterium — 76
22. Spirochetes — 82
23. Mycoplasma — 88
24. Miscellaneous — 90
25. Rickettsiaceae — 94
26. Chlamydiae — 98
27. General Properties of Viruses — 101

28.	Bacteriophage	105
29.	Herpesviruses	108
30.	Orthomyxoviruses	114
31.	Paramyxoviruses	117
32.	Arbovirus	121
33.	Rabies Virus	124
34.	Hepatitis Virus	126
35.	Slow Virus Diseases	131
36.	Miscellaneous Viruses	133
37.	Picornaviruses	137
38.	AIDS	141
39.	Introduction to Parasitology	146
40.	Ameba	147
41.	Intestinal, Oral, and Genital Flagellates	153
42.	Cryptosporidium Parvum	157
43.	Pneumocystis Jirovecii	159
44.	Coccidia	161
45.	Malaria	163
46.	Trematodes	174
47.	Intestinal Flukes	175
48.	Cestodes (Tapeworms)	183
49.	Nematodes	186
50.	Mycology	212
51.	Superficial Mycoses	215
52.	Deep Mycoses	219
53.	Otomycosis	230
54.	Mycotic Poisoning	231
Appendices		233
Index		249

1 General Microbiology

LOUIS PASTEUR

CONTRIBUTIONS

- Techniques of sterilization
- Developed the steam sterilizer
- Established differing growth needs of bacteria
- Contributed information about anthrax, chicken cholera and rabies
- Developed live vaccines – chicken cholera and anthrax
- Coined the term VACCINE.

KOCH'S POSTULATES

Microorganism accepted as causative agent of an infectious disease only if following conditions are satisfied:
- Bacterium should be constantly associated with lesion of disease
- Should be possible to isolate bacterium in pure culture from lesions
- Inoculation of such pure culture into suitable laboratory animals should reproduce lesions of disease
- It should be possible to reisolate the bacterium in pure culture from the lesions produced in experimental animals
- Specific antibodies to the bacterium should be demonstrable in serum of patients suffering from the disease.

QUELLUNG REACTION

- One of the methods to demonstrate capsule besides Indian ink negative stain
- It is a serological method as capsular material is antigenic
- Method:
  - Suspension of capsulated bacterium is mixed with its specific anticapsular serum
  - Examined under microscope
  - Capsule become prominent and swollen due to increased refractivity
- Use for typing *S.pneumoniae*.

Bacterial Spore

- Ability of few bacteria to form highly resistant resting stages
- The process of formation of spore is known as sporulation
- Not a method of reproduction and are endospores
- Occurs during vegetative growth after depletion of exogenous nutrients.
- Process:
  - Appearance of clear area at one end of cell which becomes opaque to form fores
  - Developed spore has nuclear body that are surrounded by spore coat
  - Followed by thick spore cortex which again enclosed by tough spore coat
  - Some have additional covering exosporium.
- Position: Central, terminal or subterminal
- Sporulation helps bacteria to survive in unfavorable states
- When favorable conditions occur they germinate.
- Demonstration
  - Forespore stained readily
  - Developed spore stained by modification of Zeil-Neelsen technique.
- Destruction: Autoclaving at 120 °C for 15 minutes.

Bacterial Growth Curve

- When a bacterium seeded in suitable liquid medium and incubated. Growth pattern follows definite course.
- Phases are
  - Lag phase
  - Log phase (exponential)
  - Stationary phase
  - Phase of decline

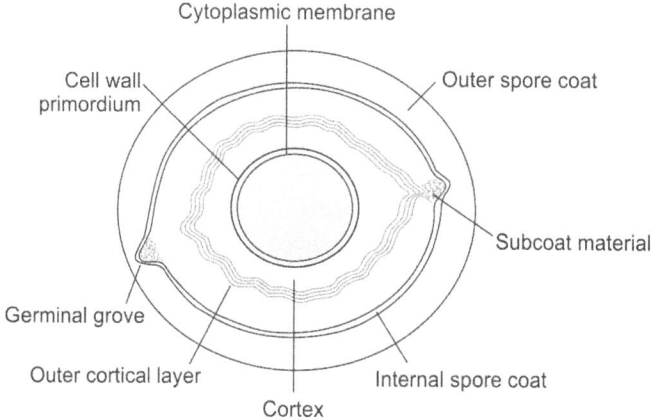

Fig. 1.1: Diagrammatic representation of a bacterial spore

LAG PHASE

- Immediately after seeding
- No appreciable ↑ in count but ↑ in size
- Time required for adaptation to new environment
- Necessary enzymes and intermediates produced
- Maximum cell size achieved at end
- Duration depends on
- Species
- Size of inoculum
- Nature of culture medium
- Environmental factors (e.g. temperature).

Log (Exponential) Phase

- Increase in cell number exponentially on geometric progression
- Log of count vs time graph–straight line
- Cells are smaller and stains uniformily.

Stationary Phase

- Division stops due to depletion of nutrients and accumulation of toxic products
- Progeny formed: Cells die
- Viable count stationary: An equilibrium is achieved between forming and dying cells
- Sporulation occurs.

Phase of Decline

- Population decrease due to cell death
- Reasons → Nutritional exhaustion
    Toxin accumulation
    Autolytic enzymes.

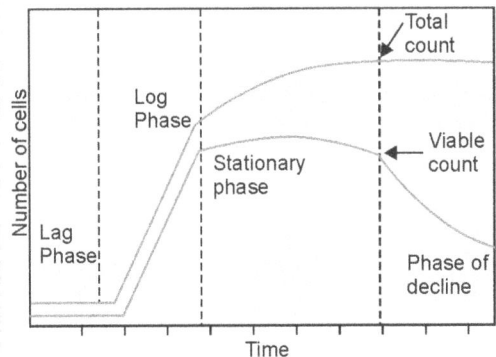

Fig. 1.2: Bacterial growth curve. The viable count shows the lag, log, stationary and decline phases. In the total count, the phase of decline is not evident

2. Sterilization and Disinfection

STERILIZATION

Process by which an article, surface or medium is freed of all living microorganisms either in the vegetative or spore state.

DISINFECTION

Destruction or removal of all pathogenic organisms or organisms capable of giving rise to infection.

Sterilizing Agents

Physical Agents	Chemical Agents
Sunlight	Alcohol
Drying	Aldehydes
Dry heat	Dyes
Moist heat	Halogens
Filtration	Phenol
Radiation	Gases

- Sunlight: Due to ultraviolet rays and heat rays.
- Drying: Since bacterial cell wall contain more water, unreliable.

HEAT

- Most reliable method of sterilization.
- Mechanism of action: Protein denaturation, oxidative damage and the toxic effect of elevated levels of electrolytes.
- Thermal death time: Minimum time required to kill a suspension of organisms at a predetermined temperature in a specified environment.

Dry Heat

Flaming

- To sterilize inoculating loop or wire, tip of forceps and searing spatulsa.
- Held in Bunsen flame till they become hot.

Incineration
- Used for sterilization of contaminated cloth, animal carcasses and pathological materials.

Hot Air Oven
- Most widely used method of dry heat sterilization.
- Mechanism of action: Hot air is a bad conductor of heat and its penetrating power is low. Then oven is heated by electricity with heating elements in wall of chambers. Materials arranged so as to free circulation of air in between the objects.
- Temperature and holding time:
    - 160 °C × 1 hr–Glassware, culture swabs, liquid paraffin and all glasses.
    - 150 °C × 2 br–Fine cutting instruments of ophthalmic surgery.
- Sterilization control:
    - Biological–Spores of nontoxigenic of clostridium tetani.
    - Chemical–Browne's tube.
    - Physical–Thermocouple.

Moist Heat

Temperature Below 100 °C

Pasteurization
- To sterilize milk.
- Heated either 63 °C for 30 minutes (Holder method) or 72 °C for 15–20 seconds (Flash process) followed by cooling quickly to 13 °C or lower.

Inspissation
- Used for sterilization of Lowenatein-Jensen and Lo-efflers serum slope.
- 80–85 °C × Half hour on three successive days.

Temperature At 100°C

Tyndallization
- Used to sterilise media containing sugar/gelatin.
- 100 °C × 20 minutes × 3 successive days.

Autoclave (Temperature above 100°C)
- Sterilization using steam under pressure.
- Mechanism: Water boils when its vapor pressure equals that of surrounding atmosphere. When steam comes contact with a surface it give heat to that surface.
- Holding time: 121°C × 15 minutes.
- Two types of autoclave: Gravity displacement and high volume vacuums.
- Working.

```
Sufficient water is added to cylinder and materials to be sterilized is kept on tray
                                    ↓
                           Autoclave is heated
                                    ↓
Lid is srewed tight and discharge tap open Adjustment of safety valve to required pressure
                                    ↓
         Steam-air mixture is allowed to escape till all air has been escaped
                                    ↓
                         Raise the inside steam pressure
                                    ↓
   When the desired steam pressure is reached, Safety valve opens and excess steam
                                    ↓
                                 Escapes
                                    ↓
                       From this holding period calculated
                                    ↓
                   Heater turned off and autoclave is cooled
                                    ↓
                           Discharge tap is opened
```

- Defects
  - Air discharge is inefficient.
  - No facility for drying.
- Sterilization control
  - Physical control – Thermocouple
  - Chemical control – Browne's tube
  - Biological control – Bacillus stearothermophilus.

Filtration

- Uses:
  - To sterilize heat labile fluids
  - To isolate pathogens from water
  - To purify water
- Commonly used filters 4
  - Membrane filter – most commonly used
  - Seitz filter
  - Sintered glass filter- prepared by heat fusing finely powdered glass particles.

Radiation

- Nonionizing radiation
  - Infrared radiation – Syringes and Catheters
  - UV – Entryways, operation theaters, laboratories
- Ionizing radiation
  a. To sterilize plasters, syringes, swabs, catheters, metal foils.

Cold Sterilization

- The process in which sterilization I carried out at low temperature
- Agents used: X-rays, Gamma rays, Cosmic rays, Chemicals, Radiation, Membranes
- Materials sterilized – Plastics, catheters, syringes, fabric, metal foils.

CHEMICAL AGENTS

Antiseptics: Chemical disinfectants which can be safely applied on skin and mucus membranes and are used to prevent infection by inhibiting bacteria.

Alcohols

- Ethyl alcohol and isopropyl alcohol (70%)
- Concentration used – 60–90% in water
- Use: Skin antiseptics.

Aldehydes

- Gluteraldehyde: Concentration is 2% optimum concentration.
  Use: Corrugated rubber, anesthetic tubes, face masks, metal instruments.
- Formaldehyde: Concentration is 10% formalin.
  Use: Sterilizing instruments and heat sensitive catheters, Fumigating operation theaters.

Phenols

1. Phenol 2. Lysol 3. Dettol
   Use: Treatment of wounds, nontoxic skin antiseptics, general disinfectants.

Gaseous disinfectants

1. Ethylene oxide 2. Formaldehyde gas 3. Betapropionolactone 4. Chlorine

Surface acting agents

1. Acetyl trimethyl ammonium bromide 2. Benzalkonium chloride

3. Culture Media and Methods

■ TYPES OF CULTURE MEDIA

- Solid media, liquid media, semisolid media
- Aerobic media, anaerobic media
- Simple media, complex media, synthetic media, semisynthetic media, special media.

Special Media

- Enriched media
- Enrichment media
- Selective media
- Indicator media
- Transport media
- Sugar media.

Liquid Media

Uses

- For obtaining bacterial growth from blood.
- For preparing bulk cultures of antigens or vaccines.

Disadvantages

- Bacteria may not exibit special characteristics
- Difficult to isolate different types of bacteria, e.g. nutrient broth, alkaline peptone water.

Solid media

- Bacteria have distinct colony morphology when cultured, e.g. cooked cut potato (earliest media), Agar, Peptone.

Simple media

- Nutrient broth – Peptone + meat extract + NaCl + Water.
- Nutrient Agar – Nutrient broth + 2% Agar.
  Increasing concentration of agar to 6% prevents swarming.

SPECIAL MEDIA

1. Enriched Media
- Substance like blood, serum/egg added to basal media.
- For growth of bacteria which are more extracting in nutrient needs, e.g. a. Brain – heart infusion agar Broth: for typhoid. b. Blood-agar.
- Consists of blood, agar and peptone.
- Example for enriched, indicator, nonselective and differential medium.
- To differentiate *grampositive cocci* based on hemolysis.
- Alpha hemolysis – greenish yellow discoloration around colony.
- Beta hemolysis – clearing around colonies.
- Gamma hemolysis – no change in medium. c. Chocolate agar
  - By heating a mixture of sheep red cells and nutrient agar.
  - RBC disrupted released contents Hb, hemin (X), NADC (factor V), e.g. H. influenza, Niesseria, Moraxella.

2. Enrichment Media
- Liquid media
- In mixed culture, bacterium to be isolated overgrown by unwanted bacteria
- Normally nonpathogenic species overgrows
- Substance that have stimulating effect on bacteria to be isolated and inhibitory effect on unwanted is incorporated into medium, e.g. Selenite F- Broth – dysentery bacilli and Tetrathionate broth – for typhi and paratyphi.

3. Selective Media
- When above substance is incorporated into solid medium.
- Greater number of required bacterial colonies are produced, e.g. Desoxycholate Citrate for dysentery bacteria
  - TCBS for vibrio
  - Thayer martin for Neisseria
  - Lowenstein- Jensen medium for Mycobacterium tuberculosis.

4. Indicator Media
- Medium which has indicator which change color when bacteria grows, e.g. Wilson blair medium – Salmonella typhi and Mcleod's medium – Pottasium tellurite to tellurium, Diphtheria bacilli.

5. Differential Media
- Has substance incorporated in it which about differing characteristics of bacteria, e.g. McConkey agar
  - Differentiate → Lactose fermenters – pink colonies
  - Nonlactose fermenters – colorless colonies.

6. Transport Media

- Delicate organism that cannot withstand time taken for transporting the specimen to laboratory, e.g. Stuart's media: nonnutrient soft agar gel that contain reducing agent and charcoal for enterococci.
    - 'Buffered Glycerol saline – for enteric bacilli'.

Anaerobic Media

- To grow anaerobic organisms, e.g.
    - Robertson's cooked meat medium
    - Thioglycollate medium
    - Sabouraud dextrose agar.

Aerobic Culture Methods

- Streak culture (Surface plating)
- Lawn or carpet culture
- Stroke culture
- Stab culture
- Pour plate culture
- Liquid culture.

ANAEROBIC CULTURE METHODS

Culture Methods

- Strict anaerobes like clostridium tetani form growth if only Oxygen tension < 2 mm Hg.

1. Mcintosh – Fildes anaerobic jar

- Most reliable and widely used.
- Parts:
    - Stout glass/metal jar with metal lid of air tight screws.
    - Two tubes with taps – one inlet and one outlet.
    - Beneath lid – two terminals that can be connected to electric supply which is connected to palladinised asbestos.
- Working:
    - Inoculated culture plates are placed inside the jar in medium in bottom half of plates.
    - Outlet tube connected to vaccum pump and air inside is evacuated.
    - Inlet tube to hydrogen supply – terminals connected to electric supply.
    - Palladinised asbestos acts as catalyst and residual oxygen reacts with hydrogen.
    - Aluminium pellets coated with palladium – in gauze sachet suspended from lid of jar act as catalyst at room temperature.

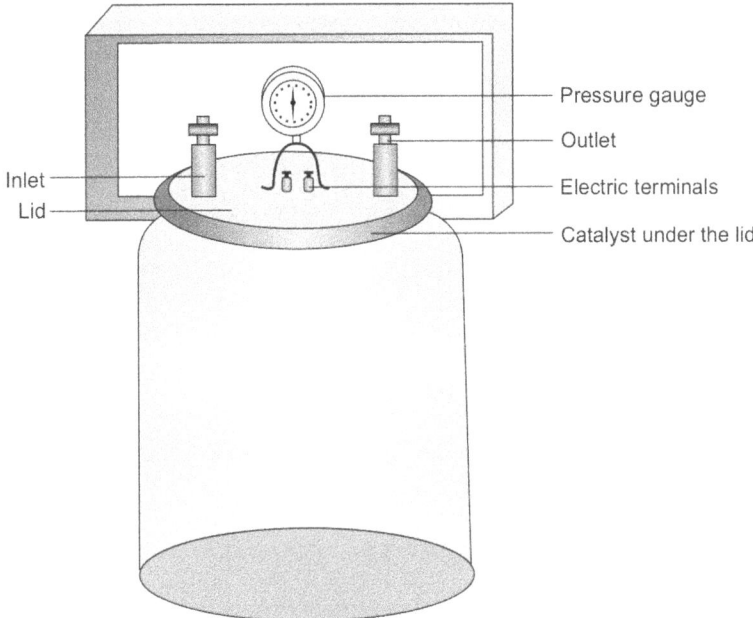

Fig. 3.1: Mcintosh and fildes anaerobic jar

2. Gaspak
- Method of choice for anaerobiosis
- Disposable envelope containing chemicals which generate hydrogen and carbon dioxide on addition of water
- It is simple and effective, eliminating the need for drawing a vacuum and adding hydrogen.

3. Prereduced anaerobic system (PRAS)
- For fastidious anaerobes.

4. Anaerobic chamber (glove box)

5. Robertson's cooked meat medium
- Most widely used fluid medium for culture of anaerobes
- Fat free minced cooked meat in broth
- Unsaturated fatty acids take up oxygen, reaction catalysed by hematin in meat and sulphydryl compounds bring about reduced oxidation reduction potential
- Saccharolytic species – Pink
- Proteolytic species – Black.

6. Other methods
- Reducing agents – 1% glucose, 0.1% ascorbic acid
- Broth – Smith Noguchi medium.
- Thioglycolate broth.

4. Bacterial Genetics

■ TRANSMISSION OF GENETIC MATERIAL

Transformation
- Takes place through the agent of free DNA.

Transduction
- Transfer of portion of DNA from one bacterium to another via bacteriophage.
- During assembly of phage inside infected bacteria packing error occurs.
- Portion of bacterial DNA is incorporated into phage nucleic acid.
- When one bacterium infect other DNA transfer is effected.
- 'Most common mechanism of gene transfer'.

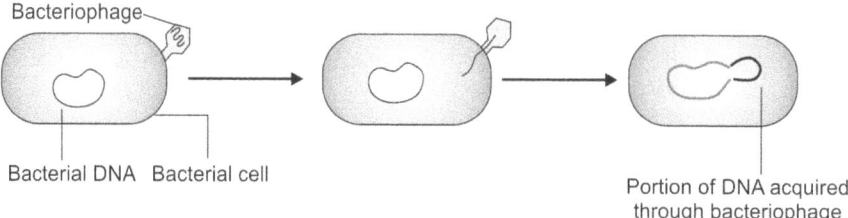

Fig. 4.1: Mechanism of gene transfer

- Types
  - Generalized: When it involves one segment of donor DNA
  - Restricted: When bacteriophage transducts only a particular genetic trait
- Most mechanism of gene transfer
- Any bacterium for which phage exist show transduction.

Lysogenic conversion
- Phage DNA is incorporated into host chromosome as prophage
- Replicates synchronously with bacterial DNA and transferred to daughter cell → lysogene
- Prophage imparts new characteristics for daughter and host bacterium → lysogene/phage conversion
- Toxigenecity in Corynebacterium diphtheria.

Conjugation

- Male/donor bacterium mates or makes physical contact with female/recipient bacterium
- Usually plasmid are frequently transferred
- Maleness is determined by presence of plasmid that encodes for specialized fimbria
- Plasmid replicates and copy transferred through pilus to recipient
- Recipient attains donor status and affects females
- Plasmid termed as fertility factor
- Then as Transfer factor when several plasmids identified.

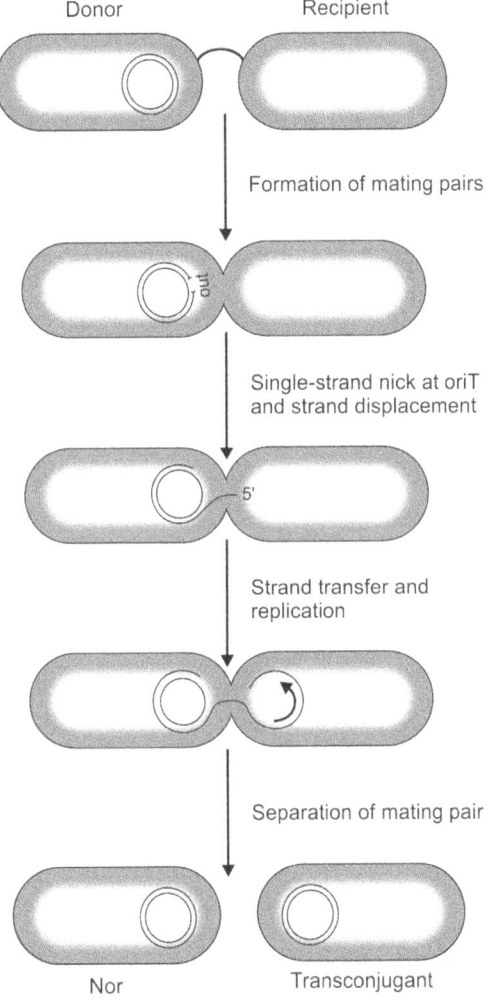

Fig. 4.2

F factor

- Contain genetic information necessary for sex pilus
- Cell having F factor → F⁺ cells mate with F⁻ cells
- F factor can be integrated into host chromosomes so called episome

- Episome can transfer chromosomal gene into recipient with high frequency (Hfr cells), following conjugation with Hfr, F⁻ rarely becomes F⁺.

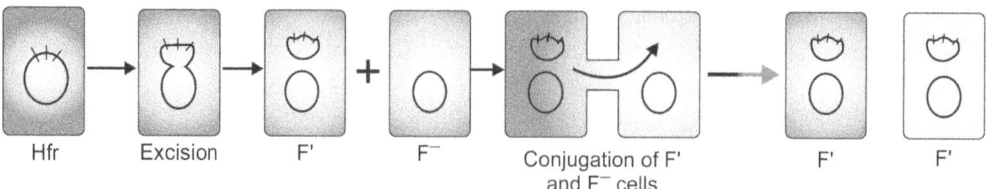

Fig. 4.3: Sexduction. The integrated F factor of an Hfr cell may revert to the cytoplasmic state. During excision some host genes may be incorporated in the F' factor (F). When an F' cell mates with F⁻ cell, the host gene is transferred to the recipient

- Hfr is reversible, when it occurs, f factor carries some chromosomal gene – F prime (F⁺).
- F⁺ cell mates recipient → transfer chromosome gene along with F factor → Sexduction.

Resistance Transfer Factor

- Plasmid that leads to spread of multiple drug resistance
- Example Shigella against pseudomonas
- Resistance is transferred by conjugation
- Mechanism of drug resistance – Transferable, episomal/Infectious drug resistance
- 2 components – Resistance Transfer factor + r determinant drug resistance combinely termed as R factor
- R factor can have several 'r' determinants
- Sometimes RTF dissociate form r determinant host cell remain drug resistant but not transferable
- In normal gut drug resistance inhibited by:
  - Anaerobic condition
  - Alkaline pH
  - Gram-positive anaerobic bacteria.

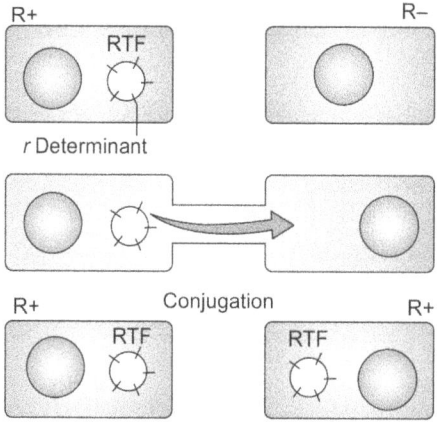

Fig. 4.4: Transferable drug resistance. The R+ cell carries the R factor, consisting of the RTF and r determinants. Its transfer to a sensitive R– bacterium converts the recipients into a resistant R⁺ cell

Mechanism of Drug Resistance in Bacteria

- Bacteria acquires resistance by mutation and method of gene transfer.
- Mutation:
  - Stepwise resistance achieved by series of small set mutation.
  - One step.

Clinical significance

- Resistance is of great importance in TB.
- It treated with streptomycin alone → initially dies → resistant mutant appears.
- 2 drug given, kills resistant mutants.

Mutational drug resistance	Transferable drug resistance
• One drug resistance at one time	• Multiple drug resistance
• Low degree resistance	• High degree resistance
• Overcome by high drug dose	• High dose ineffective
• Drug combination can prevent	• Drug combination ineffective
• Do not spread	• Spread to other species
• Mutant may be defective	• Not defective
• Low virulence	• High virulence

Transposable Genetic Element

- Ability of a DNA segment to move around in cut and paste manner between chromosomal and extrachromosomal DNA
- These DNA are Transposons or Jumping genes
- Mode of transfer is Transposition
- Transposons
  - DNA segment with one or more gene at center
  - Two ends carrying inverted repeat sequence of nucleotides
  - Complementary to each other but in reverse order
- Each strand can form loop carrying gene and double stranded stem formed by hydrogen bond
- Imparts new characteristics
- Cannot replicate its own
- No homology with transposable gene of donor and recipient gene.

5 Infection

INFECTION

Lodgement and multiplication of parasite in the host.
- Primary infection: Initial infection of parasite with a host.
- Secondary infection: New parasite sets up an infection in a host whose resistance is lowered by pre-existing infectious disease.
- Cross-infection.
- Iatrogenic infection: Physician induced infection.
- Nosocomial infection: Hospital acquired infection.

SOURCE OF INFECTION

a. Humans
- Carrier: Person who harbors pathogenic microorganism without suffering any ill effect.
- Convalescent carrier: One who recovered disease and continue to harbor the pathogen.
- Temporary carrier: Less than 6 months.
- Chronic carrier: For several years.

b. Animals

c. Insects

d. Soil, water and food

Method of Transmission
- Contact
- Inhalation
- Ingestion
- Inoculation
- Insects
- Congenital.

BACTERIAL CELL WALL

Pathogenecity – Factors
- Pathogenecity
- Virulence

- Exaltation
- Attenuation

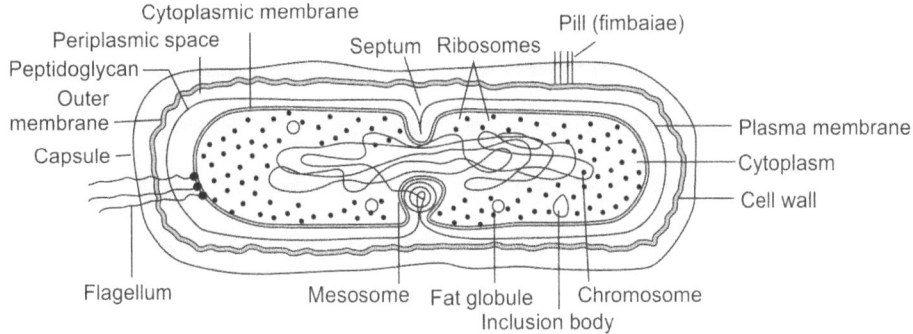

Fig. 5.1: Bacterial cell wall

Virulence determinants

- Adhesion
- Invasiveness
- Plasmids
- Bacteriophage derived
- Communicability
- Toxigenicity.

Exotoxins	Endotoxins
• Proteins	• Lipopolysaccharide
• Heat labile	• Heat stable
• Actively secreted by cell	• Form part of cell wall
• Diffuse into surrounding medium	• Do not diffuse into surrounding media
• Separate from culture	• Obtained only by cell lysis
• Action enzymic	• Nonenzymatic reaction
• Specific pharmacological effect	• Nonspecific effect
• Specific tissue affinities	• Nonspecific tissue affinity
• Active in very minute dose	• Active in very large dose
• Action specifically neutralized by antibody	• Neutralization by antibody ineffective

Types of infectious diseases

- Localized, generalised
- Superficial, Deep
- Bacteremia: Presence of bacteria in blood
- Septicemia: Bacteria and its toxins in blood
- Pyemia: Septicemia with multiple abscesses in internal organs
- Epidemic: That spreads rapidly, involving many person in an area at a same time
- Endemic: Constantly present in a particular area
- Pandemic: Epidemic that spread through more than one continent
- Prosodemic: Creeping epidemics that evolve at a slower rate, e.g. cerebrospinal fever.

6 Immunology

- Term referred to the resistance exhibited by the host towards injury caused by microorganism.

TYPES

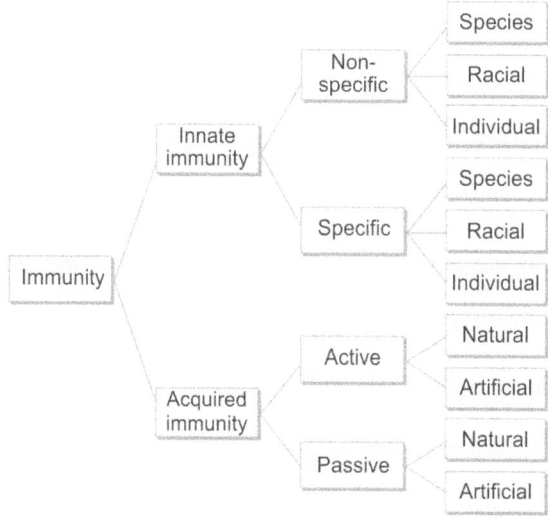

ADAPTIVE IMMUNITY

- Defined as resistance an individual acquires during life by recognizing and selectively eliminating specific foreign molecules.
- Four characteristic features—Antigen specificity, Diversity, Immunologic memory, Self/non-self recognition.

Active Immunity

- Resistance developed by an individual as a result of an antigenic stimulus
- Active functioning of hosts immune apparatus leading to synthesis of antibodies and immunologically active cells
- During development of immunity, negative phase seen as antigen combines with pre-existing antibody
- Once developed, long lasting and response is greater in secondary exposure
- Active immunity associated with immunologic memory

- More effective and better protection than passive
- Two types: Natural and Artificial.

Natural
- Due to clinical or inapparent infection of microbe
- Immunity may be life long (chickenpox) or short lived (common cold)
- Immunity following bacterial infection less permanent than viral infection
- Premunition: Immunity to reinfection lasts only as long as infection persists (as in syphilis).

Artificial
- Induced by vaccines

TYPE	BACTERIAL	VIRAL
Live	BCG	OPV (Sabin)
Killed	Cholera vaccine	Injectable polio vaccine
Subunit	Typhoid VI antigen	Hep B vaccine
Bacterial products	Tetanus toxoid	

Passive Immunity
- Resistance transmitted passively to a recipient in a retrograde form
- No antigenic stimulus; instead preformed antibodies are administered
- No latent period of action
- No negative phase
- No secondary type response occurs as in active immunity instead elimination occurs
- Less effective than active immunization
- Two types: Natural and Artificial.

Natural
- From mother to baby
- Ig A in milk (colostrum) and Ig G through placenta.

Artificial
- Administration of antibodies
- Hyperimmune sera of human or animal cell origin is used
- Used for prophylaxis and therapy
- Convalescent sera and pooled human gammaglobulin contains antibodies against some viral hepatitis
- Indication
  - Emergency or temporary protection
  - To suppress active immunity when it becomes injurious
- Combined immunization
- Both active and passive immunization
- This is to provide protection till active immunity starts.

Antigens

- Specifically as molecules that interact with the immunoglobulin receptor of B-cells or T-cells when complexed with MHC.
- Attributes of Antigenicity:
  - Induction of an immune response (Immunogenicity).
  - Specific reaction with antibodies (Immunological reaction).
- Types of Antigen:
  - **Complete antigen**: Able to induce antibody and specifically react with them in an observable manner.
  - **Haptens**: Cannot induce antibody themselves. Specifically react with antibody. Can be immunogenic by combining with large molecular carrier.

Epitope

- Present on antigen
- Smallest unit of antigenicity
- Consist of 4 or 5 amino acids or monosaccharides
- Having a specific chemical structure, electric charge and steric configuration
- 2 type
  a. Sequential or linear epitope: single linear structure.
  b. Conformational epitope: having tertiary structure.

Paratope

- Combining site on antibody corresponding to epitope.

Biological Classes of Antigens

- Based on the ability to induce antibody formation, antigens classified into

T-cell independent antigen	T-cell dependent antigen
Does not need participation of T-cells for response of B- cell to antigen	Need participation of T-cell
Structurally simple	Structurally complex
Too little dose , nonimmunogenic	
High dose, results in immunological tolerance	Immunogenic over wide range and do not cause tolerance readily

ANTIBODIES (IMMUNOGLOBULINS)

- Antigen binding glycoproteins
- Heterodimer
- Have 2 identical light chains and 2 heavy chain
- Chains are connected by disulphide bridge
- Variable region determines binding with antigen
- Light chains : Kappa and Lambda in the ratio 2:1
- Antibodies are of 5 types depending on heavy chain.

Ig G

- Most abundant 80% of total Ig
- Highest concentration in plasma
- Distributed approximately equally between extravascular and intravascular compartment
- Its catabolism varies with its serum concentration
- When its level is raised it is catabolized rapidly
- When in case of hypo gamma globulinemia, Ig G given for treatment will be catabolized slowly
- Longest half life (23 days)
- Four types : Ig G1, Ig G2, Ig G3, Ig G4
- Participates in most immunological reaction such as complement fixation test, precipitation and neutralization of toxins and viruses
- Only antibody to be transferred transplacentally.

Ig A

- Provide local immunity
- 10–13% of total serum
- Activates alternate complement pathway
- Exists as monomer/polymer
- In serum exist as monomer
- In secretions exist as dimer-secretory Ig A
- 2 Types: Ig A1 and Ig A2
- Important line of defense against salmonella, vibrio, neisseria, polio, influenza and reovirus.

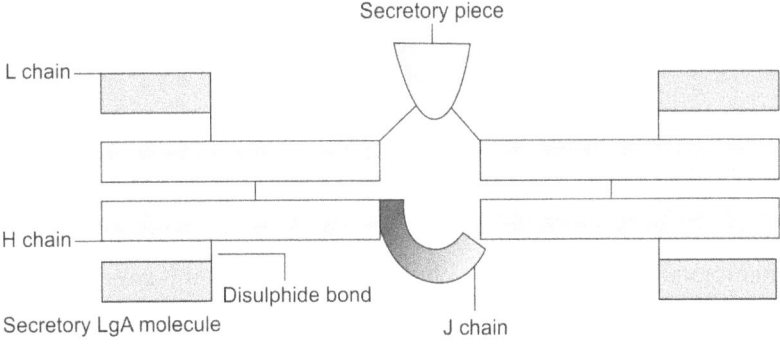

Fig. 6.1

Ig M:

- 5–8% of serum Ig
- Half-life: 5 days
- First immunoglobulin produced in response to antigenic stimulus

- Millionaire molecule
- 80% intravascular
- J chain present
- First immunoglobulin to be synthesized by neonates
- Short lived, disappier earlier than Ig G
- Also act as secretory Ig after Ig A
- 2- mercapto ethanol selectively destroys Ig M
- Not transported across placenta, so presence in fetal serum indicates intrauterine infections.

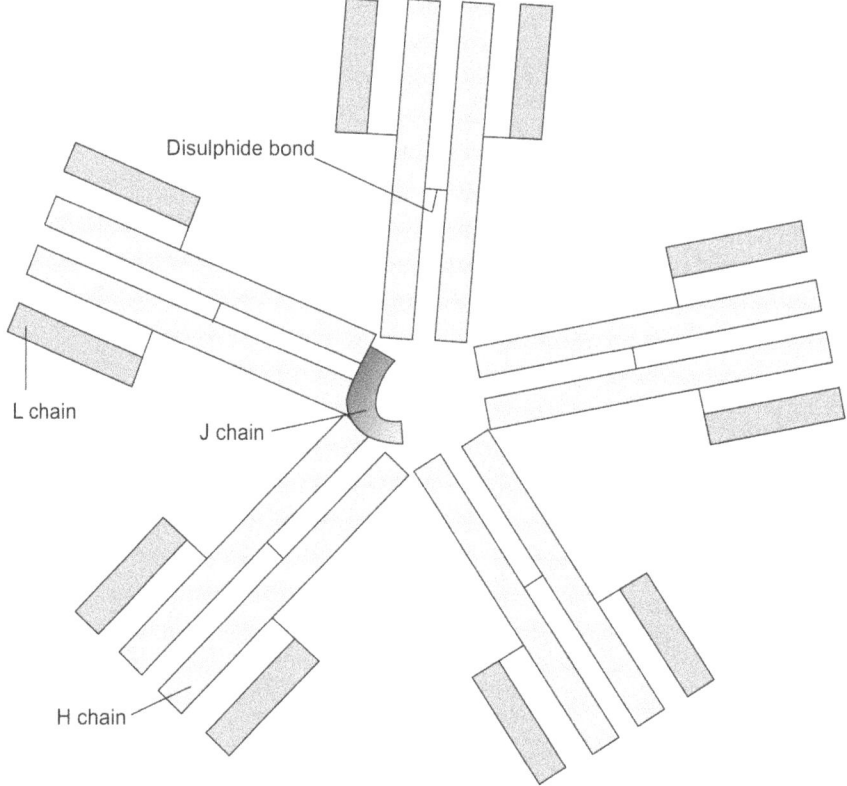

Fig. 6.2: Ig M Molecule

Ig D
- 1–3% of serum Ig
- Half-life: 3 days
- Major membrane bound immunoglobulin on unstimulated B-cell.

Ig E
- Mostly extravascular
- Least abundant in serum
- Homocytotropic: human Ig E fix to human cell
- Heat labile
- Induce mast cell degranulation and type 1 hypersensitivity reaction
- No placental crossing, no complement fixation.

Monoclonal antibodies

- Derived from a single clone and specific for single epitope
- Previously produced by hybridoma technique
- Role in therapeutic, imaging and diagnostic purpose.

Uses

- Diagnosis of hepatitis, influenza, herpes
- Isolation of a particular substance (interferon)
- Imaging and therapy
- Research purposes

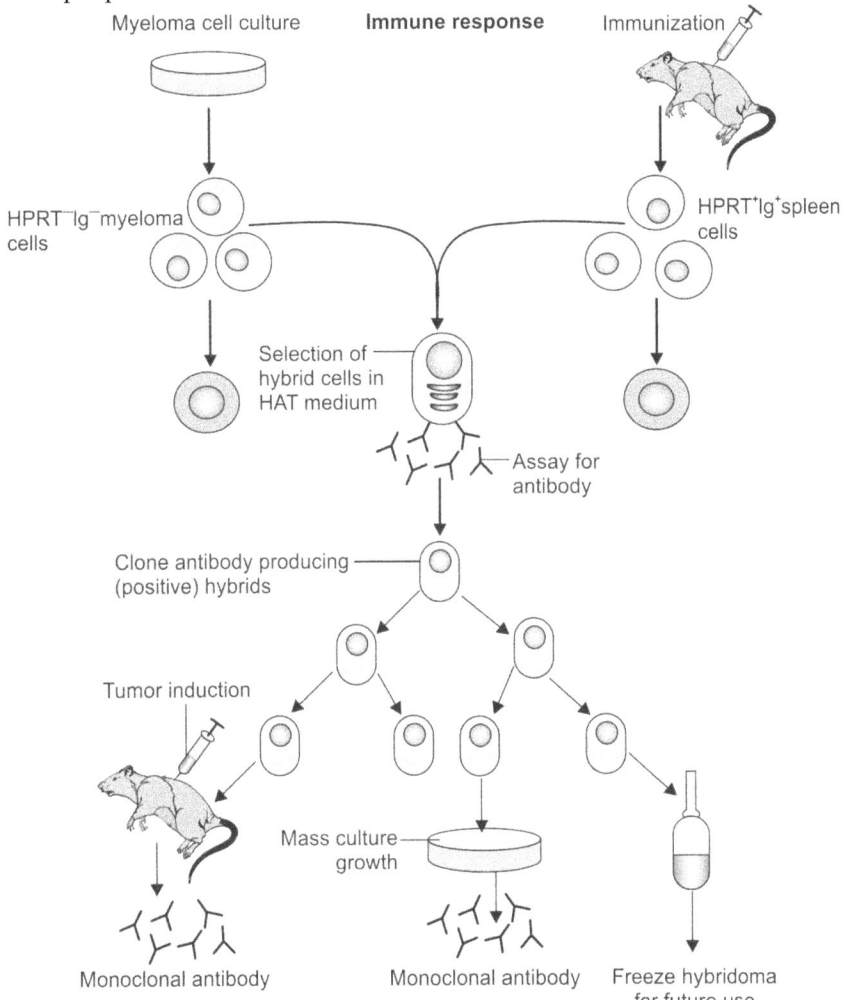

Fig. 6.3: Monoclonal antibody production by hybridoma

Multiple Myeloma

- Malignancy of antibody producing plasma cell
- Excess of light chain: Bens jones proteins
- Coagulation at 50 °C and dissolves at 70 °C.

In Short
- Ig G protects body fluids
- Ig A protects body surface
- Ig M protects bloodstream
- Ig E mediates reaginic hypersensitivity
- Ig D recognition molecule of B-cell.

ANTIGEN ANTIBODY REACTION

- The reactions between them are important and has application in body, in laboratories, screening population, etc.
- *In vitro* reactions are known as serological reactions
- The reaction occur in three stages—primary, secondary and tertiary
- Antibody is also called agglutinin and corresponding antigen as agglutinogen.

Precipitation Reactions
- Precipitation: When a soluble antigen combines with its antibody in the presence of electrolytes at a suitable temperature and pH
- Flocculation: Instead of sedimenting, precipitate remains suspended as floccules
- 3 phases:
   a. Prozone phenomenon: Caused by excess antibody
      Inhibition of lattice formation
      Cause failure of visible reaction
   b. Zone of equivalence: Antigen and antibody are in optimum proportions
      Visible reaction seen
   c. Post zone phenomenon: Presence of excess antigen in test system

Applications
- Forensic application in identification of blood and other stains
- Testing for food adulterants
- Grouping of streptococci by Lancefield technique
- The VDRL test for syphilis
- Test toxigenicity in diphtheria bacilli.

Immunodiffusion
- Here precipitation occurs in a gel
- Reaction is visible as a distinct band of precipitation, which is stable
- Many modifications are present today
   — Single diffusion in one dimension
   — Double diffusion in one dimension
   — Single diffusion in two dimension
   — Double diffusion in two dimension
   — Immune electrophoresis.

Electroimmunodiffusion
- The development of precipitin lines can be speeded up by electrically driving the antigen and antibody with diffusion using various methods:
  - Counter immune electrophoresis
  - One dimensional single electroimmune diffusion
  - Two dimensional electrophoresis.

Agglutination Reaction
- When particulate antigen is mixed with its antibody in presence of electrolytes at a suitable temperature and pH- they are clumped and agglutinated
- More sensitive than precipitation for detection of antibodies
- Three types:
  a. Slide agglutination: Blood grouping and cross matching
  b. Tube agglutination: In serological diagnosis of typhoid, brucellosis, typhus fever
  c. Heterophile agglutination test: Weil-Felix test
  Streptococcus MG agglutination test Paul bunnel test

Coomb's Test
- **Principle:** When incomplete antibodies are mixed with antigen positive red cells, they coat the cells but does not agglutinates. When such cells are washed free of other proteins and treated with rabbitantiserum against human gamma globulin, get agglutinated.
- Two types
  a. Direct : Occurs in vivo: When infant RBC mixed with coomb's serum, agglutination occurs, e.g. hemolytic disease of newborn
  b. Indirect: Occurs in vitro: Used in autoimmune hemolytic anemia, brucellosis.

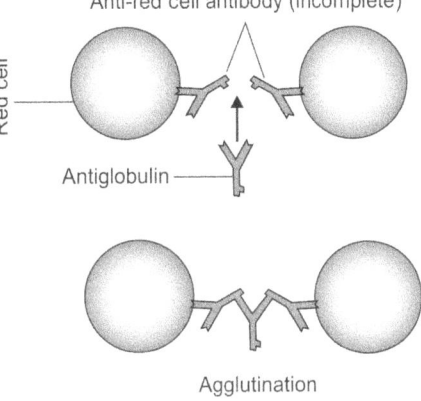

Fig. 6.4: Coomb's test

Passive Agglutination Test
- Here soluble antigens is attached to surface of carrier particles
- It is possible to convert precipitation to agglutination tests
- Commonly used carrier particles: RBC, latex particles or bentonite, e.g.
  - Hemagglutination: Rose waaler test used in rheumatoid arthritis
  - Latex agglutination test: ASO, CRP, RA factor, HCG determination
  - Co-agglutination test: Here antibody adsorbed to carrier particles
    For diagnosis of Legionella, S. pyogens, etc.

Complement Fixation Test
- **Principle:** Ability of antigen antibody complex to fix complement is made used. Sensitive test (0.04 mg antibody and 0.1 mg antigen is enough)
- Involves 2 steps and 5 reagents
- Reagents are antigen, antibody, complement, sheep erythrocytes and amboceptor

- **Procedure:**
  - Antigen is soluble or particulate.
  - Antiserum is heated (50 °C) and inactivated.
  - Complement is from guinea pig serum which is stored in lyophilized frozen state.
- **Step 1**
  - Antigen + test serum + complement.
- **Step 2**
  - To above step hemolytic system is added.

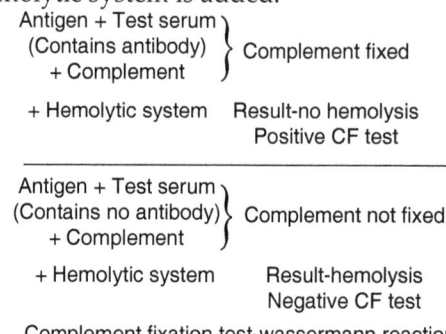

Complement fixation test-wassermann reaction

Indirect Complement Fixation Test
- Done in case of sera that do not fix guinea pig complement
- First step same as above
- Before second step standard antiserum that fixes complement is added
- If antibody present antigen must be used in first step
- Does not able to fix the complement in second step
- Here lysis indicates positive result.

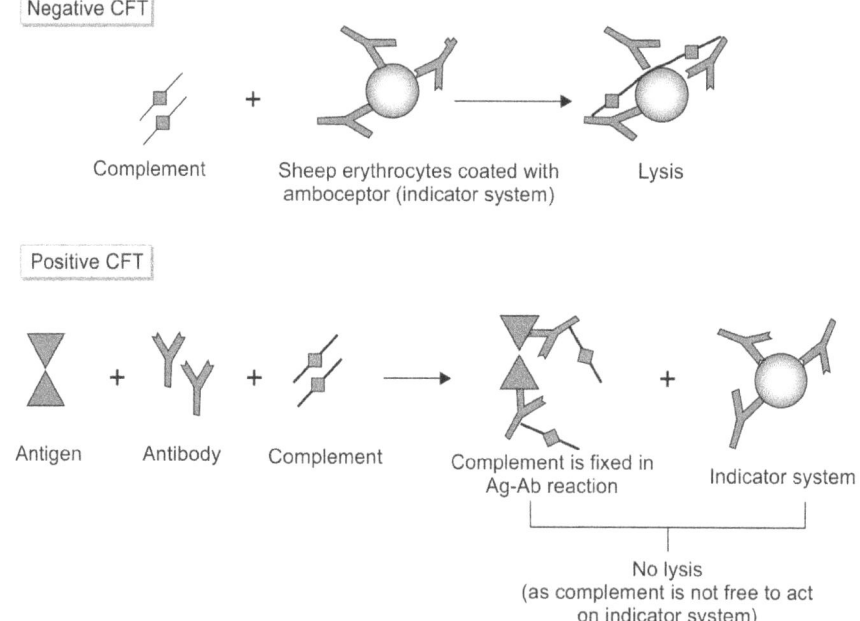

Fig. 6.5: Complement fixation test

ELISA
- Enzyme linked immune sorbent assay
- Here immunosorbent is used as absorbing material for antigen or antibody like polythene, cellulose or agarose.

Procedure
- Microtiter plate are coated with antibody specific to antigen
- After thorough washing samples are added and incubated (37 °c for 2 hours).
- Wells washed and antiserum of antigen labelled with alkaline phosphatase added
- Wash again and para nitro phenyl phosphate added and look for yellow color
- If color develops the reaction occurred and is positive and vice versa.

Types
- Sandwich ELISA: antibody coated plate
- Indirect ELISA
- Competitive ELISA: Conjugate (antibody to antigen) labelled is added and looked for color. If positive no color develops as conjugate gets washed away
- Capture ELISA
- Cylinder/cassette ELISA.

Uses
- HIV detection
- Infectious disease: Hepatitis, EBV, CMV, Dengue Ig G
- Rotavirus detection and enterotoxin in E.coli in feces
- Syphilis Ig G/Ig M, H.pylori Ig G
- Food toxins, adulterants
- Human allergen.

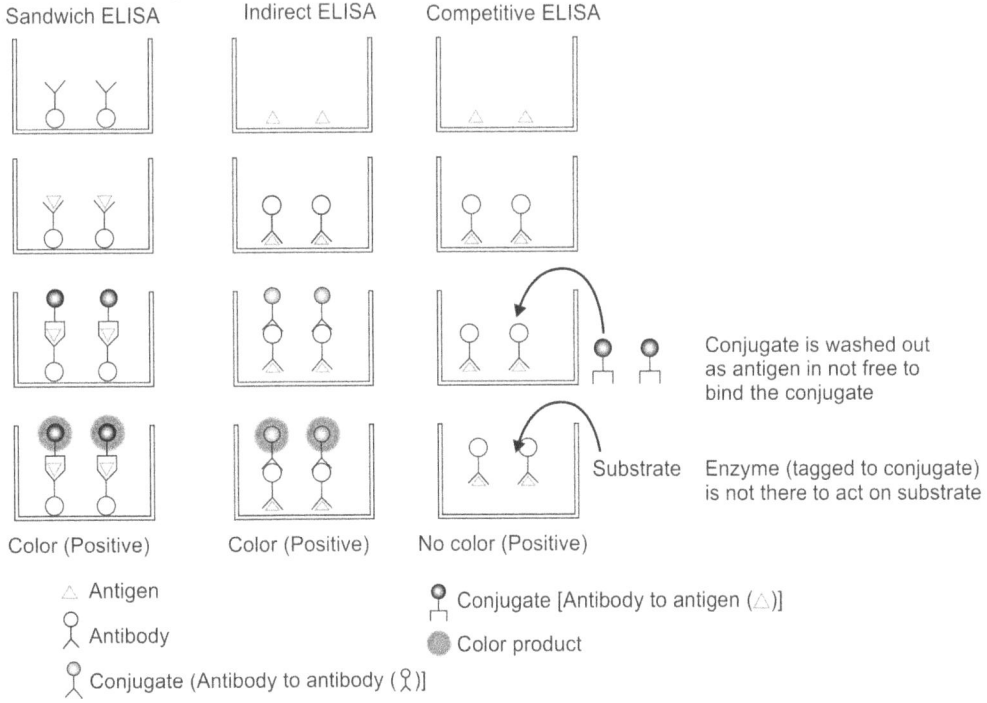

Fig. 6.6: Enzyme linked immunosorbent assay (ELISA)

Immunofluorescence

Direct Immunofluorescence Test

Identification of bacteria, viruses or other antigens using specific antiserum labelled with a fluorescent dye.

Indirect Immunofluorescence

- Here no separate fluorescent conjugates to each antigen is required
- Drop of test serum is placed on smear of organism and washed well to remove all free serum and only antibody globulin remains which is then treated with fluorescent labelled antiserum to human gamma globulin
- Fluorescent dye exposure reacts with antibody globulin and examined under UV light
- Seen as bright object against a dark background.

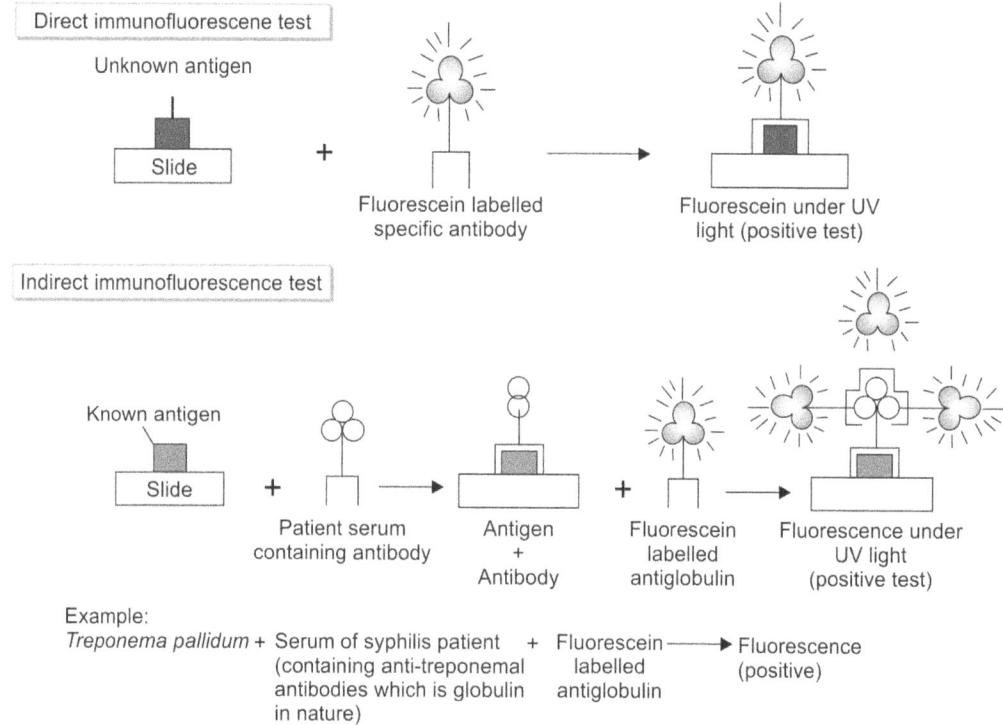

Fig. 6.7: Direct and indirect immunofluorescence test

Other Reactions

- Neutralization test
- Opsonization
- Radioimmunoassay
- Chemiluminescence immunoassay
- Western blot test.

HYPERSENSITIVITY

- Inappropriate immune response to a sensitized antigen resulting in significant tissue damage or even death.
- Injurious consequence in a sensitized host cell following contact with specific antigens.

Coomb's and Gell Classification

Based on pathogenesis

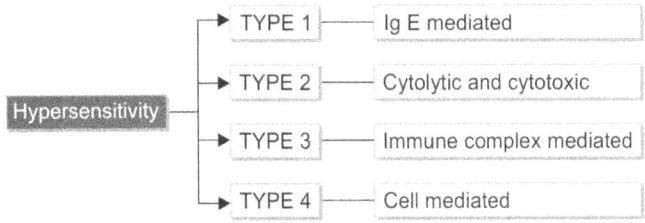

Immediate hypersensitivity	Delayed hypersensitivity
Appears and react rapidly	Appear slowly
Induced by antigen by any route	Induced by antigen only by skin contact
Antibody mediated	Not antibody mediated
Passive transfer possible with serum	Passive transfer possible only with T-cells or transfer factor
Desensitization easy but short lived	Desensitization difficult but long lived
Includes type 1, 2 and 3 hypersensitivity	Type 4 hypersensitivity

Type 1 Hypersensitivity

- Ig E dependent
- Allergen: an antigen that cause allergy
  Genetic predisposition, e.g. Proteins: Serum, Vaccines
  Plant Pollens
  Drugs: Penicillin, Sulfa drugs, Local anesthetics
  Food: Nut, Sea food, Egg, Peas, Milk.

Mechanism

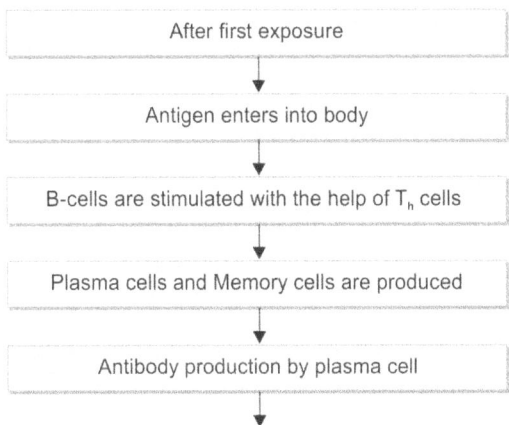

Contd...

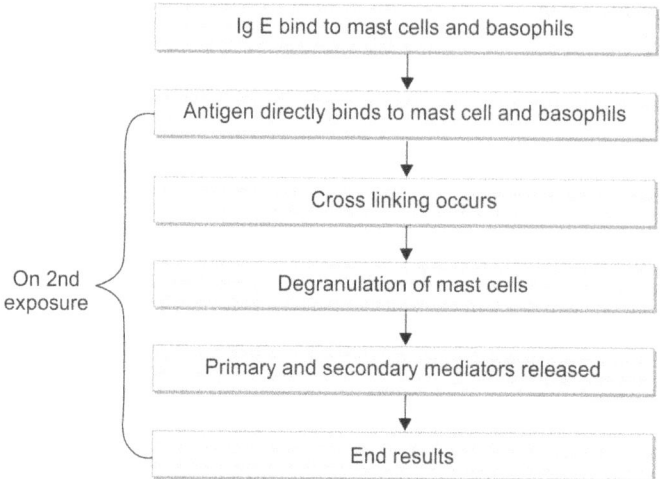

- Primary mediators: Histamine, heparin, serotonin
- Secondary mediators: Leukotrienes, cytokines, prostaglandins
- End results: Smooth muscle contraction, increased vascular permeability, vasodilation.

Effects

Systemic
- Called anaphylaxis
- Acute potentially fatal systemic form caused by venom from bee, drugs such as penicillin.

Local
- Known as atopy
- Chronic, recurrent, nonfatal, localized, and inherited
- Affects only at site of entry of allergen, e.g. Asthma, Hay fever, Eczema, Food allergy.

Diagnosis
- Skin testing
- RIST and RAST
- ELISA.

Prevention
- Allergen avoidance
- Hyposensitivity by repeated injection of increased doses of allergen
- Immunotherapy with monoclonal antibodies
- Drug therapy (Antihistamines, Epinephrine, Steroids).

Type 2 Hypersensitivity
- Antibody mediated (antigen-antibody complex not used now)
- Cytolytic and cytotoxic
- Ig G or Ig M is produced.

Mechanism

- Antigen enters ⟶ Ig G/Ig M produced ⟶ Antigen Antibody complex
  Lysis of Antigen ⟵ Classical complements pathway activation ⟵
- Antigen enters ⟶ Antibody produced ⟶ Antigen Antibody complex
  Opsonisation by phagocytes they act as opsonin ⟵ with the help of c3b ⟵
  Ag-Ab-C3b complex is formed
- Ag-Ab complex ⟶ Attract and stimulates CD8 T-cells ⟶ Cell lysis occur, e.g.
  - Transfusion reactions
    ABO incompatibility
    Rh incompatibility
  - Drug induced hemolytic anemia
    Penicillins, cephalosporins, streptomycin
  - Grave's disease and Myasthenia gravis.

Type 3 Hypersensitivity

- Immune complex mediated
- Ag – Ab forms an immune complex with the help of complement
- Normally this complex is destroyed in spleen otherwise it get deposited in blood vessels, synovial membrane of joints, glomerular basement membrane of kidney, choroid plexus of brain.

Mechanism

- Ag- Ab complex
  ↓
- Classical complement pathway activation ⟶ Immune complex formation
- C3a, C4a, C5a are anaphylotoxins which activate mast cells and cause vasodilation
- C3a and C5a attracts neutrophils, which fails to phagocytose large immune complex
- The frustrated phagocytes release enzymes that damage local tissues.

Effects

Local

- Immune complex deposits only at site of entry
- Arthus type reactions: Erythematous and edematous intense neutrophilic infiltration, e.g. Farmers lung, Erythema nodosum leprosum, Intrapleural arthus type pneumonitis or alveolitis.

Systemic

- Immune complex deposits in tissue where filtration of plasma occurs (kidney, arteries, joints).

Type Three Associated Diseases

Autoimmune	SLE, Rheumatoid Arthritis, Good Pasteur's Syndrome
Drug Reactions	Penicillin, Sulfa Drugs
Infectious Disease	Post Streptococcal Glomerulonephritis

Type Four Hypersensitivity
- Also known as delayed hypersensitivity
- Cell mediated
- Occurs 24–72 hours after antigen contact
- No antibody involved.

Type 5 Hypersensitivity
- Here the antibody activates the receptor sites and enhances the activity of the cell, e.g. Long Actin thyroid stimulator (LATS).

Mechanism
- Involves Two phases

Sensitizing phase

Antigen + Antigen presenting cell + MHC II presented to CD4 T-cells
↓
T-cells are sensitized

Effector phase
Second contact with same antigen

Sensitized T_h cell take up antigen
T_h cell produce cytokines
↓
Recruitment of macrophage
↓
Phagocytose antigen and cause tissue damage

NOTE: Here delay is due to time taken for T-cells to produce procytokines, macrophage recruitment and subsequent reactions.

TYPES
- **Tuberculin type:**
  - Tuberculin antigen is injected intradermally on flexor aspect of forearm
  - After 48–72 hours induration formed
  - Size > 10 mm test
  - < 5 mm test negative
  - 5–9 mm equivocal
- **Granulomatous type:**
  - Granuloma is formed
  - Bacteria: M.tuberculosis, M.leprae, Brucella
  - Fungi: Histoplasma, Cryptococcus, Candida
  - Parasite: Leishmania
  - Virus: Herpes simplex, Smallpox, Measles.
- **Contact dermatitis:**
  - Skin contact with certain substance causes hypersensitivity e.g. metals, hair dyes, poison ivy, picryl chloride, nickel salt.

Antigen complex with skin protein ⟶ captured by Langerhans cells
Same as above ⟵ Cytokines ⟵ Activation of T_h cells ⟵

AUTOIMMUNITY

- Structural and functional damage produced by auto antibodies and immuno competent T-lymphocytes against own normal tissues.

General Features of Autoimmune Disease
- Elevated Ig levels
- Demonstrate auto antibodies
- Deposition of Ig/immuno complex at sites
  - Chronic, nonreversible
  - Definite female preponderance 3:1.

Mechanism of Autoimmunity
- Physical
- Chemical
- Biological
- Mutation
- Molecular mimicry and cross reacting antigen
- Hidden or sequestrated antigens (lens proteins and sperm antigens)
- Polyclonal B-cell activation
  - Nonspecific activation of B-cell by chemical, drugs, enzymes, bacteria, viral and parasites
  - Emergence of forbidden clones
  - T and B cell defects
  - MHC II molecules over expression.

Classification

Hemolytic	Localized organospecific	Systemic
Autoimmune hemolytic anemia	Hashimoto thyroiditis	Rheumatoid arthritis
Idiopathic thrombocytopenic purpura	Grave's disease	SLE
	Addison's disease	Good pasteur's syndrome
	Autoimmune orchitis	
	Myasthenia gravis	
	Pernicious anemia	

Pathogenesis
- Either humoral or cell mediated immunity against self-antigen.
- Autoantibodies are more compared to cellular autosensitization.
- Type 2 cytotoxic.

Therapy
- All diseases are chronic
- Immunosuppressive drugs
- Thymectomy
- Plasmapheresis
- Synthetic blocking peptides competing with autoantigen to bind to MHC
- Monoclonal antibody
- Tolerance to autoantigens oral administration.

7 Streptococcus

- Gram-positive cocci arranged in chains
- Most important is Streptococcus pyogenes
- Classification of Streptococcus — Lancefield and Griffith
- They are catalase negative.

Antigenic structure

- Carbohydrate antigen
- Protein antigen – M, T, R proteins
- Hair like pili.

Toxins and other virulence factors

- Hemolysins
- Streptolysin O } Responsible for lysis
- Streptolysin S
- 'Pyogenic Exotoxin' **(Dick, Scarlatinal toxin)** – Super antigens responsible for **scarlet fever**
- Streptokinase
- Streptodornase
- NADase
- Hyaluronidase.

Pathogenicity

Suppurative

- Respiratory infections
  - Tonsillitis or pharyngitis – most common
  - Caused by virulent group A streptococci
  - More common in older children and adults
  - May spread to form otitis media, mastoiditis, quinsy
  - Ludwig's angina and suppurative adenitis
- Skin and soft tissue infections
  - Erysipelas
  - Impetigo

- Cellulitis
- Necrotizing fasciitis
- Others
  - Abscesses in internal organs such as brain, lungs, liver and kidneys.

Nonsuppurative – Post streptococcal sequelae
- Occurs 1–3 weeks after acute infection due to antibody reactions
- Two important sequelae—acute rheumatic fever and acute glomerulonephritis.

	Acute Rheumatic fever	Acute glomerulonephritis
Infection of	Throat	Throat or skin
Prior sensitization	Essential	Not necessary
Immune response	marked	Moderate
Penicillin prophylaxis	Essential	Not indicated
Complement level	Unaffected	Lowered
	Like an autoimmune reaction	Like type III hypersensitivity reaction
	Cross link between streptococcus and heat tissue	Ag-Ab complex (immune)
		Deposit in glomerular membrane

Lab Diagnosis
- Specimen: Throat swab, pus swab or exudates
  Serum in nonsuppurative lesions
- Microscopy: Gram staining
- Culture: Blood agar - β hemolytic colonies, catalase negative
- Transport medium: Pike's medium
- Identification: Rapid diagnostic test kits are available
Bacitracin sensitivity
- Serology
- *ASO titer:* Antistreptolysin O titer
  - > 200 indicative of prior infection
    High levels in a/c rheumatic fever and AGN.
- Anti-DNAase B estimation—acute Glomerulonephritis
- Streptozyme test.

Prophylaxis
- Long-term administration of penicillin in children who have early signs of rheumatic fever.

Treatment
- Sensitive to Penicillin – G.
- Most are sensitive to erythromycin.

CAMP test
- For group B streptococcus
- S. Agalactiae – important in neonatal meningitis

- On blood agar lytic Staph aureus is streaked horizontally through middle and test strains are streaked perpendicular to above line
- Arrow shaped accentuated zone of hemolysis occurs in case of Group B streptococci near the vertical streak.

STREPTOCOCCUS PNEUMONIAE

- Commonly known as pneumococci
- Gram-positive diplococci
- Normal inhabitants of the human upper respiratory tract
- Capsulated, capsule enclosing each pair
- B-Bile solubility
- O-Optochin sensitive
- P – Polysaccharride capsule
- I – Inulin fermentation.

Antigenic Structure

- Capsular polysaccharide specific soluble substance (SSS)
- Nucleoprotein
- Somatic 'C' carbohydrate antigen.

Toxins and virulence factors Virulence depends on

- Capsular polysaccharide: Prevent phagocytosis
- Pneumolysin: Cytotoxic and complement activating properties
- Autolysins
- Quellung reaction: Capsular swelling (mentioned earlier).

Pathogenecity and clinical features

Normal inhabitants of nasopharynx
↓
Aspiration of nasopharyngeal secretions
↓
Multiply and penetrate bronchial mucosa ← Compromise of normal defense by viral infection
↓
Spread through lung along lymphatics
↓
Lobar pneumonia and Bronchopneumonia

- Infection of the middle ear, heart, peritoneum and joints
- Acute tracheobronchitis, empyema
- Acute exacerbations in chronic bronchitis
- Meningitis and suppurative lesions.

Most Important infections are Pneumonia and Meningitis.

Lab Diagnosis

- Specimen: Sputum, CSF, blood, urine
- Microscopy: Gram staining: Gram-positive diplococci seen inside polymorphs and also extracellularly
- Culture – blood agar: After incubation small glistening, dome shaped colonies with an area of green discoloration (alpha hemolysis) around them. 'draughtsman' or carrom coin appearance
- Reactions: Bile solubility and Optochin sensitivity
- Antigen detection: Demonstration of SSS in CSF
  - Detection of polysaccharide Ag in urine by immunochromatography
- Biomarkers: CRP testing
  - Procalcitonin: Elevated in invasive areas
- Molecular methods: PCR.

Prophylaxis

- Polyvalent polysaccharide vaccine:
  Dose: 0.5 ml, Route: s/c or IM, Site: anterolateral thigh
- Schedule: Three doses at ≥ 6 weeks apart and one booster at 15–18 months
- Adverse reactions: Fever, local pain, soreness, malaise
- Contraindication: Anaphylaxis after previous dose
- Storage 2–8 °C, do not freeze.

Treatment

DOC: Parenteral pencillin
Resistant cases: Third gen. cephalosporins
Life-threatening cases: Vancomycin.

8 Staphylococcus

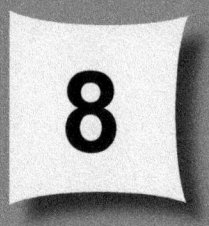

- Staphylococcal infections are most common among bacterial infections
- Gram-positive cocci occurring in grape like clusters
- Nonmotile, non-sporing
- Mainly produce localized pyogenic lesions.

Common-pyogenic staphylococcal infection
- Skin and soft tissue: Folliculitis, furuncle, abscess, common wound infection, impetigo, paronychia
- Musculoskeletal: Osteomyelitis, arthritis, bursitis
- Respiratory: Tonslilitis, pharyngitis, sinusitis, otitis, bronchopneumonia, lung abscess
- CNS: Meningitis, abscess
- Endovascular: Bacteremia, septicemia, pyemia
- Urinary: Urinary tract infection.

Common toxin mediated staphylococcal diseases
- Food poisoning
- Toxic shock syndrome
- Scalded skin syndrome.

Pathogenesis: Two types of disease

Infection: Bacteria gain access to damaged skin *Intoxication:* by bacterial toxins
↓
Colonize
↓
Evade host defense
↓
Multiply and cause damage

Virulence factors
- Cell associated polymers:
  - Polysaccharide peptidoglycans
  - Teichoic acid
  - Capsule polysacharide.

- Cell surface proteins (clumping factor)
    a. Bound coagulase
    b. Protein A:
        Binds to Fc terminal of IgG molecule leaving the Fab region free. This property is involved in co-agglutination reaction.
- Extracellular enzymes
- Coagulase: Brings about clotting of human or rabbit plasma, Acts with coagulase reacting factor binding to prothrombin which converts fibrinogen to fibrin.
    - Lipid hydrolase
    - Hyaluronidase
    - Nuclease.

Toxins
- Cytolytic toxins: hemolysins: $\alpha, \beta, \gamma, \delta$
    leucocidin
- Enterotoxin:
    - Responsible for manifestation of staphylococcal food poisoning
    - Source of infection is usually a food handler who is a carrier
    - Acts directly on autonomic nervous system
- Epidermolytic toxin.

Toxic Shock Syndrome
- By toxic shock syndrome producing S. aureus (type 1 most often responsible)
- Multisystem disease characterized by fever, hypotension, myalgia, vomiting, diarrhea, mucosal hyperemia and erythematous rash
- TSST are super antigens which are potent activator of T lymphocytes and stimulate very large number of T cells without epitope specificity
- Associated with tampon related infections, surgical wound infections
- Super antigens are β restricted T cell mitogens.

Laboratory Diagnosis
1. Specimen: Depends on type of lesion, e.g. pus from suppurative lesion, sputum for respiratory infections and for carriers nasal swab
2. Microscopy: Gram-positive cocci arranged in clusters
3. Culture
    - Nutrient agar: Large opaque golden yellow colonies with oil paint appearance
    - Blood agar: Hemolytic
    - Mac conkey agar: Pink colonies due to lactose fermentation
    - Selective media: Salt-milk agar, Ludlam's, Robertson cooked meat medium

4. Identification-catalase positive
   - Coagulase test- two types

Tube coagulase test	Slide coagulase test
• 0.1 ml of young broth culture + 0.5 ml of human plasma	
• EDTA, heparin or oxalate as anticoagulant	• Done in slide
• +ve and -ve controls kept	• Prior to test, check for auto agglutination by using normal saline
• Tubes incubated in a water bath • If +ve - plasma clots and does not flow when tube is tilted	

   - Antibiotic sensitivity test
   - Typing
- Serological Test.

Treatment

- Benzyl penicillin is most effective if sensitive
- But 80% are resistant, so Cloxacillin is DOC
- Drug resistance is common due to:
  - Production of beta lactamase
  - Development of tolerance to pencillin: Only inhibited, not killed
  - Alteration in penicillin binding proteins
  - Methicillin is the first to produce resistance.

Methicillin resistant staph. Aureus (MRSA)

- Mainly associated with hospital infection due to presence of certain strains in hospital environment called hospital strains
- Treated by vancomycin and linezolid
- Rx of carrier by local application of antibiotics such as mupirocin.

9. Neisseria

- Contains gram-negative, aerobic, nonmotile, oxidase positive intracellular diplococci.
- Two important pathogens
  1. Neisseria meningitidis
  2. Neisseria gonorrhea.

NEISSERIA MENINGITIDIS

Mainly cause cerebrospinal meningitis and meningococcal septicemia.

Pathogenesis

- Due to the endotoxin, lipopolysaccharide
- Human nasopharynx is only reservoir of meningococcus
- Meningitis:
  - Droplet transmission
  - Nasopharynx →Perineural sheath of olfactory nerve→cribriform plate → subarachnoid space
  - On reaching CNS, it establishes a suppurative lesion on the surface of spinal cord, as well as base and cortex of brain
  - Some develop chronic or recurrent meningitis.

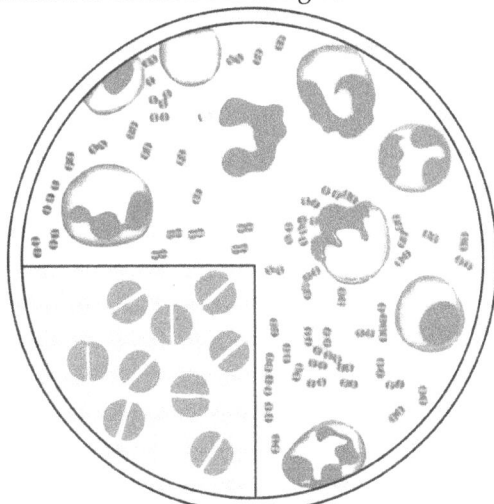

Fig. 9.1: N. Meningitidis in cerebrospinal fluid. Inset: Enlarged view showing flat adjacent sides of the cocci

- Meningococcemia:
  - Present as a/c fever with chills, malaise and prostration
  - Typical petechial rash occur early in the disease
  - Fulminant meningococcemia→formerly called Waterhouse Friderichsen Syndrome, is a fatal condition characterized by Shock, DIC and Multisystem failure

Lab Diagnosis

- Specimen: CSF, blood, skin scrapings from petechial lesions, nasopharyngeal swab (for detection of carriers)
- Examination of CSF : CSF pressure increased. Turbid with large number of pus cells.
  - For bacteriology CSF is divided into 3 portions
  - First portion: Centrifuged and gram stained. Seen as diplococci inside polymorphs or extracellularly. Supernatent contains meningococcal antigen demonstrated by latex agglutination or counter immunoelectrophoresis using meningococcal antisera
  - Second portion: Inoculated on blood agar or chocolate agar. Colony identified by morphology and biochemical reactions
  - Third portion: Incubated overnight after adding equal volume of glucose broth. Subcultured on chocolate agar
- Blood Culture
- Serology: detection of antibodies.
- Molecular diagnosis by PCR
  - Selective medium: Thayer Martin medium
  - Biochemical reaction: Oxidase +ve, maltose and glucose fermented.

Treatment

DOC: IV Penicillin G, third generation cephalosporins.

Prophylaxis

Chemoprophylaxis – By Rifampicin or Ciprofloxacin

Vaccines – monovalent and polyvalent vaccines containing capsular polysaccharides of groups A, C, W 135 and Y.

N.GONORRHEA

- Exclusively human disease caused by N. gonorrhea
- Source of infection: Human carrier or patient
- Mode of infection: Veneral.

Antigenic Properties

- Surface structures include:
  - Pili – for attachment to host cell and inhibit phagocytosis
  - Outer membrane proteins
- Endotoxin
- IgA1 protease.

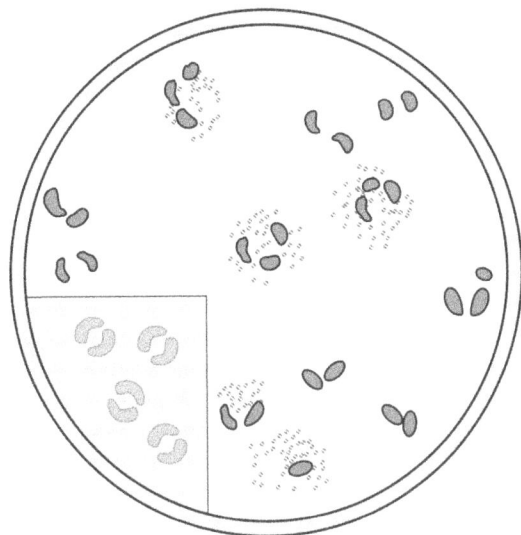

Fig. 9.2: Gonococci in urethral pus. Inse: Enlarged view to show kidney-shaped cells with adjacent surfaces concave

Pathogenicity
- Adhesion of gonococci to urethra or other mucosal surfaces→penetration to intercellular space→subepithelial connective tissue.

In men: disease starts as a/c urethritis with mucopurulent discharge:
- Infection can extend to prostate, seminal vesicles and epididymis
- Water can perineum: Periurethral spread of infection causing abscess and multiple discharging sinuses
- In women: mainly involves urethra and cervix uteri
- Vagina usually spared due to stratified squamous epithelium
- Acidic pH of secretions
- Infection may spread to Bartholin's gland, endometrium and fallopian tubes
- **Fitz-Hugh-Curtis syndrome:** Peritonitis may develop with perihepatic inflammation
- Disseminated gonococcal infection
- Proctitis in both sex
- Conjunctivitis
- Blood invasion from primary site and lead to metastatic lesions
- Ophthalmia neonatorum: Not sexually transmitted
- Gonococcal bacteremia.

Lab Diagnosis
- Specimen: Discharge, urethral swab, endocervical swab. Morning drop of secretions is examined. Urine may be examined in absence of urethral discharge
- Microscopy: Intracellular gram-negative cocci. Kidney shaped cells

- Culture: Transport medium – Stuart's medium.
  - Blood agar
  - Chocolate agar
  - Muller Hinton agar
  - Growth identified by morphology and biochemical reactions
  - Selective medium-Thayer Martin agar
- Serology: Precipitation test, CFT, Passive agglutination, Radio immunoassay
- Molecular method: PCR.

Treatment

- Ceftriaxone 125 mg single IM dose, Ciprofloxacin 500 mg. If resistant to ciprofloxacin, ceftriaxone 125 mg IM, 1g Azithromycin single dose.
- PPNG: Penicillinase producing Neisseria gonorrhea. Drug resistance common due to beta-lactamase production.

Gonococci	Meningococci
• Not normal flora	• Present in normal flora
• Source: cases	• Source: patient or carriers
• Sexually transmitted	• Droplet transmission
• Glucose only fermented	• Glucose +maltose fermented
• Drug resistance: plasmid mediated	• Drug resistance rare
• No vaccine	• Vaccines available
• Not capsulated	• Capsulated

- Both are oxidase +ve, intracellular gram –vediplococci.

Non Gonococcal Urethritis

- Caused by organisms other than gonococci
- Gonococci cannot be demonstrated
- Caused by Chlamydia trachomatis, Ureaplasma urealyticum and Mycoplasma hominis
- Viruses: CMV and Herpes viruses
- Protozoa: Trichomonas vaginalis
- Fungi: Candida albicans
- It can also be part of Reiter's syndrome: Urethritis + arthritis + Conjunctivitis
- Samples collected same as in gonococci
- Lab diagnosis: Gram staining will not demonstrate any organisms. Only pus cells.

10. Vibrio Cholera

VIBRIO CHOLERA

- Gram-negative, curved bacilli with polar flagellum
- Grows best in alkaline pH
- Needs 0.5–1% NaCl for its growth
- Darting motility is seen

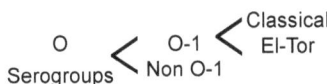

- Both classical and El-Tor contains Ogawa, Inaba and Hikojima strain.

CHOLERA

- Acute diarrheal disease
- Characterized by profuse, painless, watery diarrhea and effortless vomiting
- Clinical features mainly due to loss of fluid
- Colorless watery fluid with mucus flecks (rice water stools).

PATHOGENESIS

- Enters orally through contaminated food and water
- Chemotaxis, motility and mucinase, proteolytic enzymes helps in crossing protective layer in small intestine
- Toxin corregulated pilus (TCP): Helps in adhesion to epithelial surface
- Hemagglutinin protease: Releases the bacteria from mucosa and helps in spreading
- Does not invade or damage cells.
- **Cholera toxin**
  - Contains A (A1 and A2) and B subunits
  - B subunit binds to GM1 ganglioside receptors in jejunum.
  - A2 fragment links A1 to B
  - Prolonged activation of adenylcyclase ⟶ Increased CAMP ⟶ out pouring of water and electrolyte to lumen.

Clinical Features
- May vary from asymptomatic form to fatal form
- Incubation period 1–5 days
- Complications: Muscular cramps, pulmonary edema, renal failure and cardiac arrhythmias.

Lab Diagnosis

Specimen
- Stool sample collected directly into a wide mouthed dry container
- Rectal swab: In case of epidemic investigations and mailing of samples to distant labs.

Transport
- Within 1 hour
- If there is any delay use Venkataraman: Ramakrishnan medium and Cary Blair medium.

Processing
- Rapid diagnosis by darting motility and its inhibition by antiserum under dark field or phase contrast microscopy.

Culture
- Direct plating: Mac Conkey agar + one selective medium (BSA or TCBS)
- Enrichment media (Alkaline peptone water and Monsurs taurocholate tellurite peptone)

Identification
- Mac Conky Agar: Nonlactose fermenting colonies
- TCBSA: Yellow colonies for V.cholera
- Motility: Darting motility
- Oxidase: Positive
- String test: Positive
- Cholera red reaction –v Positive
- Final identification using antisera: O1 antiserum
  Ogawa
  Inaba.

Treatment
- Adequate replacement of lost fluid and electrolytes
- ORS and IV fluids
- Oral tetracycline used.

Prophylaxis
- Provision of protected water supply and improvement in environmental sanitation
- Vaccines: Parenteral and oral (killed B subunit of cholera toxin and live classic, El-Tor, O-139 strains).

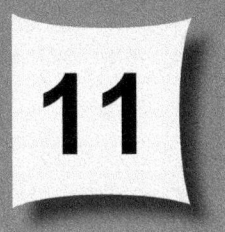

Bacillus

Spore bearing Gram-positive bacilli → *Aerobic* – Bacillus
　　　　　　　　　　　　　　　　　　Anaerobic – Clostridium

BACILLUS ANTHRACIS

Morphology
- Largest pathogenic bacteria
- Nonmotile and spore forming
- Capsulated Polypeptide capsule.

Pathogenicity
Virulence factors (mainly two)

1. *Capsular polysaccharide*
   - Inhibit phagocytosis
   - Adds to virulence
   - Sterne vaccine obtained

2. *Anthrax toxin (3 fractions)*
   a. Edema factor
   b. Protective antigen factor
   c. Lethal factor
      − Source of infection: Humans – via inhalation and ingestion of spores
No human to human transmission.

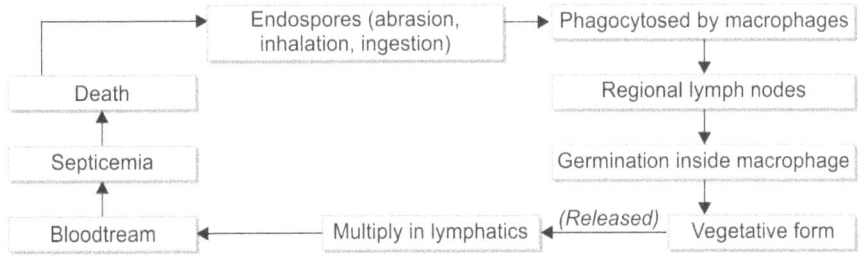

ANTHRAX

- Zoonosis
- Human anthrax – 3 types

Cutaneous Anthrax (Hide Porter's Disease)

- Most common > 95%
- Sites: Face, neck, arm, hands and back
- Hide porters disease: Common in dock workers
- Lesion: Malignant pustule.

Malignant pustule (imp short note)

Stages:

- Papule
- Vesicle
- Congestion of whole area and edema
- Satellite lesions around a necrotic area
- Covered by Eschar
- Spontaneous resolution

Pulmonary Anthrax

- Wool sorter's disease: Wool workers via inhalation from infected wool
- This is a hemorrhagic pneumonia
- Hemorrhagic necrotizing mediastinitis.

Gastrointestinal Anthrax

- Consumption of poorly cooked contaminated meat
- Enteritis with bloody diarrhea.

Lab Diagnosis

Specimen

- Cutaneous anthrax: Aspirate/swab
- Pulmonary anthrax: Sputum
- Septicaemic anthrax: Blood

Microscopy: Gram-positive bacill; Bamboo stick appearance; Central oval nonbulging spores.

Staining Techniques

- Sudan black B
- Polychrome methylene blue: Amorphous
  Purplish material around bacilli (**Mc** Fadyean's reaction)
- Immunofluorescent microscopy.

Culture

- Blood agar: Nonhemolytic colonies → Medusa head appearance
- Gelatin stab culture: Inverted Fir tree appearance
- Solid media containing penicillin: String of pearls reaction
- Selective medium: PLET medium (polymyxin, lysozyme, EDTA, Thallous acetate)

Serology: Ascoli's thermoprecipitin test.

Treatment

- Penicillin G
- Ciprofloxacin, Doxycyclin.

12 Clostridium

Gram-positive anaerobic spore forming bacilli.

Classification

Position of spores	Both proteolytic and saccharolytic	Slightly proteolytic not saccharolytic
Central or Subterminal Oval and terminal spherical and terminal	Cl.bifermentes Cl.perfringes Cl.difficle	Cl.tetani

GAS GANGRENE

- Rapidly progressive edematous myonecrosis
- Disease of war, road accidents, crush injury
- Causative agents – Cl.perfringes (main)
  - Cl.histolyticum, Cl.septicum, Cl.novyi
  - Anaerobic streptococci, E.coli, Proteus.

Pathogenesis

- Three levels
  1. Simple wound contamination
  2. Anaerobic cellulitis fasciitis
  3. Gas gangrene

  Clostridia multiply and release toxin lecithinase ⟶ ↑vascular permeability ⟶ ↑Extravasation ⟶ ↑tension ⟶ Anoxic damage

Clinical features

- Pain, tenderness, edema and crepitus due to gas formation
- Signs of toxemia
- Thin watery discharge.

Lab diagnosis

- Essentially clinical
- Laboratory investigation: Confirmational
- Specimen: Blood Films of muscle edge, tissue from necrotic areas and exudate

- Microscopy
  - Gram-positive bacilli without spore: Cl.perfringes
  - Gramstain of exudates: Scanty pus cell
  - Anaerobic streptococcal myositis (Differential diagnosis): Abundant pus cell.
- Culture
  - Aerobic and Anaerobic Blood agar
  - Robertson cooked meat medium (RCM): Turned pink (Saccharolytic).

Nagler Reaction (Lecithinase effect)

- Cl. Perfringes grown in a medium containing 6% Agar+ 5% Filde's peptic digest of sheep+ 20% human serum
- Antitoxin spread on one half of the plate
- Colonies on opposite half: Surrounded by an opacity
- Colonies on half of plate with antitoxin: No opacity due to neutralization of toxin.

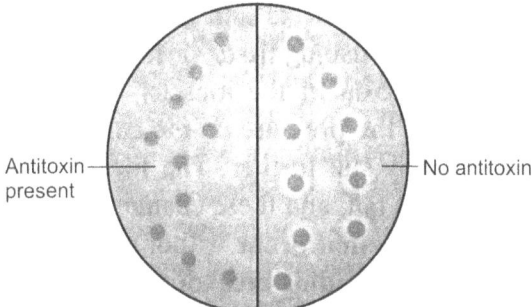

Fig. 12.1: Nagler reaction

- Identified by Morphology and culture characteristics
- Reverse c AMP test.

Prophylaxis and treatment

- Surgery – excision antibiotics – Gentamicin and amoxicillin (prophylaxis)
- Hyperbaric O_2
- Passive immunization with antigas gangrene serum.

Botulism

- Paralytic disease present in form of food poisoning
- Causative agent – Clostridium botulinum.

Pathogenecity

- Powerful neurotoxin released during cell lysis is responsible for pathogenecity
- Toxin inhibit synthesis and release of acetylcholine at NMJ or synapses – so causes flaccid paralysis
- Toxin is not digestive and absorbed from intestine in active form.

Clinical Features

- Diplopia, dysphagia, dysarthria
- Asymmetric descending paralysis
- Death due to respiratory paralysis.

Forms of Botulism

- Food borne botulism
- Ingestion of preformed toxin present in meat and meat products
- Symptoms start within 12–36 hours and include vomiting, thirst, constipation, dysphagia, dysarthria, diplopia
- Death due to respiratory failure.

Wound Botulism

- Cl.botulinum in wound produce toxin ⟶ absorbed
- Clinical features same as above except GI manifestation.

Infant Botulism

- Due to presence of spores in honey and other substances
- Clinical features include constipation, weakness, altered cry, poor oral feeding, pooling of secretions and loss of head control
- Only supportive treatment, assisted feeding. No antibiotics.

Lab Diagnosis

- Demonstration of Bacillus or toxin ⟶ Food or Feces
- Mice inoculation
- Retrospective diagnosis: Presence of antitoxin in patient serum.

13 Tetanus

- Tonic muscular spasm
- Causative agent – Clostridium tetani.

Pathogenesis

- Mode of infection: Puncture wound, surgical operations, local suppuration, septic abortion.

  Toxins → Tetanolysin
  ↘ Tetanospasmin

  Tetanospasmin → Absorbed to motor nerve endings → CNS → Block presynaptic inhibitory terminals which use glycine and GABA → Uncontrolled spread of impulse as inhibitory neurotransmitters are inhibited.

Clinical features

- Trismus (Lock Jaw)
- Spasms.

Lab diagnosis

- Sample: Bits of tissue from necrotic debris
- Microscopy: Drum stick appearance, Gram-positive organism with terminal spores.

Culture

- Blood agar swarming growth RCM – Turned black (Proteolytic)
- Gelatin stab culture – Fir tree appearance
- *In vitro* and *in vivo* tests for toxigenicity.

Prophylaxis

- Surgical, antibiotic and immunization.

Immunization

Passive immunization	Active immunization
• Tetanus antiserum from hyperimmune horse	• Toxoid
ADR: Immune elimination, hypersensitivity	• Dose: 3 doses
• Human antitetanus immunoglobulin.	1st dose: 4–6 week apart
	2nd dose: 6 months later
	Booster dose: 6 months after.

Tetanus Prophylaxis in Wound

Nature of wound	Immune	Partially immune	Nonimmune
Clean	Toxoid × 1 Toxoid × 1	Toxoid × 1	Toxoid × 3
Contaminated		Toxoid × 1 TIG antibiotics	Toxoid × 3 TIG antibiotics
Infected	Toxoid × 1 antibiotics	Toxoid × 1 TIG antibiotics	Toxoid × 3 TIG antibiotics

Treatment

- TIG: IV infusion
- Penicillin/metronidazole.

14 Enterobacteriaceae

■ COLIFORMS – PROTEUS

- Enterobacteriaceae: They are enteric pathogens which are catalase positive, oxidase negative, glucose fermenting and nitrate positive
- They grow on ordinary media and if motile it is by peritrichous flagella.

Classification

Based on their action on lactose in McConkey medium	Other classification based on family

1. Lactose fermenters
Example Escherichia, Klebsiella
2. Non lactose fermenters, e.g. salmonella, Shigella, Proteus
	1. Escherichiae
	   Genus: 1. Escherichia
	             2. Edwardsiella
	             3. Salmonella
	             4. Shigella
	2. Klebsielleae
	   Genus: 1. Klebsiella
	             2. Enterobacter
	             3. Hafnia
	             4. Serratia
	3. Proteae
	   Genus: 1. Proteus
	             2. Providencia
	4. Erwinieae
	   Genus: 1. Erwinia
	5. Yersiniae

Escherichia Coli

- Gram-negative bacillus
- Motile by Peritrichate flagella.

Antigenic structure

- O antigen (Somatic antigen): 170 types
- K antigen (Capsular antigen): 100 types
- H antigen (Flagellar antigen): 75 types

Virulence Factors

- Surface antigens: Endotoxic activity and protect from phagocytosis
    P fimbria: Plasmid mediated

Specifically bind to P blood group substance on human RBC and uroepithelial cells. Role in UTI
- Toxins – 2 types
    1. Hemolysins: Not relevant in pathogenesis.
    2. Enterotoxins: Important in pathogenesis.
- Bundle forming pilus in EPEC
- Colony forming antigen in ETEC
- Invasiveness in EIEC.

Enterotoxins

- Heat labile toxin (LT): resemble cholera toxin
- Heat stable toxin(ST): instead of c AMP, c GMP gets activated
- Verotoxin (VT) or Shiga like toxin (SLT).

Heat labile toxin

- A and B subunit
- B subunit binds to Gm 1 ganglioside receptors in intestinal epithelial cell ⟶ A gets activated ⟶ activates adenyl cyclase ⟶ c AMP↑ ⟶ diarrhea.

Clinical features

- Produce four types of clinical syndromes
    a. Urinary tract infection (UTI)
        UTI causing organisms: E. coli, Klebsiella, Proteus, Pseudomonas (catheterized patients)
    b. Diarrhea
    c. Pyogenic infections
    d. Neonatal meningitis and Septicemia.

■ UTI (ESSAY)

- Include acute urethritis and cystitis.

Culture

Screening of UTI

- Griess Nitrate Test
- Dip slide culture: Agar coated slides placed understream of urine
- Catalase: Peroxidase test
- Glucose utlization test
- TTC reduction test.

Risk factors

- Pregnancy
- Bladder outflow obstruction, e.g. BPH, Ca prostate, Urethral Stricture
- Urethral catheter
- Neurological problems, e.g. Multiple sclerosis, Spina bifida.

Asymptomatic bacteriuria: 5–7% of pregnant women have UTI without any symptoms. Such asymptomatic bacteriuria may lead to symptomatic infection later in pregnancy includes Pyelonephritis and HTN in pregnant women, prematurity and perinatal death in fetus.

Lab Diagnosis
Sample collection
- **Midstream urine sample**
  - Men: After retracting prepuce, glans penis is cleaned with wet cotton and collect the urine.
  - Women: Urine is collected after anogenital toilet using soap and water.
- **Catheter sample**
  - In cathetised patients.
  - Aspirate sample with sterile syringe needle from the proximal end of catheter after clamping and proper disinfection of catheter tube.
- **Suprapubic aspirate for children below 2 years.**

Transport: Transport specimen to lab within half an hour, if any delay refrigerate the sample or add boric acid as preservative.

Processing
- Macroscopy: Clear/Turbid
- Microscopy: Wet film examination/Gram staining Pus cells with bacteria.

Culture: Semi quantitative culture is done to know the number of bacteria/ml of urine and is done on blood agar and Mc Conkey agar.

Semiquantitative culture methods
- Standard loop method
  - Loop transfers 0.001 ml of urine is used.
  - Colony count >100 means >1 lakh bacteria/ml of urine.
- Dip slide method
- Pour plate method.

Significant Bacteriuria (Kass concept)
- If a properly collected and transported urine sample on culture contain more than 1 lakh bacteria/ml of urine is considered as significant
- Less than 10,000 bacteria/ml Contaminants.

Identification
- Blood agar for colony count
- Mc Conkey agar for differentiating LF and NLF
- Gram stain from growth – gram-negative bacteria
- Biochemical reactions
- E. Coli – G+ L+ S- M+ I+ M+ Vi- C-
- Klebsiella – G+ L+ S+ M+ I- M- Vi+ C+
- Antibiotic sensitivity tests.

Treatment
- First line drugs: Ampicillin, Cotrimoxazole, Cephalexin, Norfloxacin, Nitrofurantoin
- Second line drugs: Amikacin, 3rd generation cephalosporins, Amoxicillin – Clavulinic acid, Ciprofloxacin.

■ DIARRHEA

Five types of diarrheagenic E. coli.

Enteropathogenic E. coli (EPEC)
- Diarrhea in infants and children as institutional outbreaks and also cause sporadic diarrhea
- Different serotypes identified by slide agglutination.

Pathogenesis
- Not fully understood
- Bacilli adherent to mucosa of upper small intestine and attached to cup like projections 'Pedestals' of enterocyte membrane
- Bundle forming pili (BFP) help in adherence.

Enterotoxigenic E.coli (ETEC)
- Causes **Traveller's diarrhea**
- Endemic in developing countries among all age groups
- Severity – Mild watery diarrhea to fatal disease

    Traveller's diarrhea
    - ETEC
    - Salmonella spp
    - Cryptosporidium parvum
    - Giardia lamblia
    - Shigella
    - Campylobacter
    - Rotavirus.

Pathogenesis
- Adherence to intestinal mucosa using Colonization factor antigen (CFA)
- Produce LT or ST
- LT resemble cholera toxin.

Diagnosis: Demonstration of enterotoxin:
- *In vivo* tests
- Ligated rabbit ileal loop
- *In vitro* tests: Tissue culture, Serological tests, ELISA.

Enteroinvasive E. coli (EIEC)
- Infection resembles Shigellosis
- Pathogenesis

- Invasion - adhesion – endocytosis –endocyte vacuole –cell lysis –multiplication –spread to adjacent cells
- This E.coli is Nonlactose Fermenting, nonmotile.

Lab diagnosis

- Sereny test
- Cell penetration in HeLa or Hep-2
- VMA (Virulence marker antigen)-ELISA test.

Enterohemorrhagic E. coli (EHEC)

- Shigatoxigenic E. coli (STEC) or Verotoxigenic E. coli (VTEC).

Pathogenesis

- Target cell as capillary endothelial cell ⟶ adhesion and produces VTEC and destroy capillary endothelial cells ⟶ microangiopathy of capillaries esp. In intestinal Glomerular apparatus ⟶ cause Hemolytic uremic syndrome.
- Common strain of E. coli O 157 H7.

Lab diagnosis

- Do not ferment sorbitol: So can be differentiated from other E.coli which ferments sorbitol by using sorbitol Mc Conkey agar
- Cytotoxic effect on verocells
- Verotoxin specific ELISA
- PCR.

Enteroaggregative E. coli (EAEC)

- Persistant diarrhea in developing countries
- Stacked brick' appearance
- Pathogenesis: Shortening of villi and necrosis by a enteroaggregative toxin.

■ SHIGELLA

- Enterobacteria
- Gram-negative rods
- Nonmotile, nonsporing, noncapsulated
- Species⟶S. dysenteriae – mannitol nonfermenting
  - S. flexneri ⎫
  - S. boydii ⎬ mannitol fermenting
  - S. sonnei ⎭
- So differentiated with help of mannitol.

S. dysenteriae

- Catalase negative
- Exibit 3 types of toxic activity
- Neurotoxicity, Enterotoxicity, Cytotoxicity.

Pathogenicity
- Cause bacillary dysentery
- Minimum infective dose: 10–100 bacilli
- Mode of transmission (**5F's**-fingers, fomites, feces, food, flies)
  - Direct ⟶ via contaminated fingers
  - Fomites
  - Water
  - Food or drink contaminated with organism
  - Flies as mechanical carriers
  - Homosexuals: Gay bowel syndrome.

Invasive property
- Resemble EIEC
- Invasive property is determined by large plasmids which codes for outer membrane protein involved in invasion called 'Virulence marker Antigen' (VMA).
- Organism binds to M cells ⟶ Invade lamina propria and enterocytes ⟶ grow and induce actin polymerization ⟶ organism in neighboring cell ⟶ Cell death and inflammation ⟶ Capillary thrombosis ⟶ Necrosis of epithelium ⟶ Transverse superficial ulcer.

Exotoxin
- Shiga toxin or verotoxin
- Less important in pathogenesis
- Endotoxin: LPS of cell wall.

Bacillary dysentery
- Incubation period: 1–7 days (average 2 days).
- Onset and clinical course variable.
- Passage of stool with blood and mucus along with tenesmus and abdominal cramps.
- Fever, vomiting.
- Complications: Arthritis, toxic neuritis, Parotitis, Conjunctivitis, Intussusception (children) and hemolytic uremic syndrome.

Lab Diagnosis
- SPECIMEN: Feces
  - Rectal swabs are not satisfactory
- Transport within one hour
- If any delay use transport medium: Cary blair medium
- Processing
  - Direct microscopy: Pus cell/RBC
  - Ova/cyst/Larva

Culture
- Direct plating: MA+ one selective medium for each pathogen
- Enrichment: Selenite F broth, Tetrathionate broth

- Selective media
  - Deoxycholate citrate agar (DCA)
  - Xylose lysine deoxycholate (XLD)
- MA: Colorless colonies (Absence of lactose fermentation)
- DCA or XLD: Pale or pink colored colonies identified by biochemical reactions
- Confirmation: Slide agglutination with polyvalent and monovalent sera
- **Serology**: Not useful.

Treatment

- Uncomplicated self-limiting.
- Replenish water and electrolytes.

ENTERIC FEVER

- Caused by S.typhi and paratyphoid A, B and C.

Pathogenesis

- Infection acquired by ingestion.
- Infective dose is 10^3–10^6.
- On reaching gut → attach to microvilli of ileal mucosa → penetrate lamina propia and submucosa → phagocytosed by polymorphs and macrophages → enter mesenteric lymph node and multiply → via thoracic duct enter bloodstream → bacteria seeded in liver, gallbladder, spleen, bone marrow, lungs, kidneys and lymph node.
- Bile is a good culture medium → multipiles → discharged into intestine → Peyer's patches and lymphoid follicle → inflammation, necrosis and slough off Typhoid ulcers.

Clinical features

- Incubation period 7–14 days.
- Gradual onset with headache, malaise, anorexia, coated tongue and abdominal discomfort, diarrhea or constipation
- Step ladder pyrexia with relative bradycardia
- Soft palpable spleen and hepatomegaly
- Rose spots on skin.

Complications

- Intestinal perforation, hemorrhage and circulatory collapse
- Bronchitis or bronchopneumonia
- Cholecystitis, arthritis, abscess, periosteitis, neuritis and thrombosis.

Carriers

- Convalescent carrier: Patient who continue to shed typhoid bacilli in feces for 3 weeks to 3 months after clinical cure
- Temporary carrier: Those who shed bacilli for more than 3 months – 1 year
- Chronic carrier: Those who shed bacilli for more than a year.

Antigenic structure

- Flagellar antigen H
- Somatic antigen O
- Surface antigen V1.

Variations

- H-O variation
- Phase variation
- V-W variation
- S-R variation.

Lab Diagnosis

Specimens collected

- Blood for culture, Widal and clot culture
- Urine
- Stool
- Bone marrow.

Tests done – Based on Duration of illness

First week

- Blood culture (yield 80 – 90%).
- Antigen detection for circulating antigen (Staphylococcal Coagglutination test)
- Widal test for baseline titer.

Second week

- Blood culture (yield 70 – 80%).
- Widal test and clot culture
- Stool and urine culture.

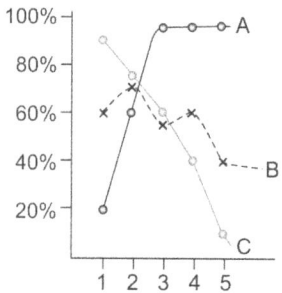

Fig. 14.1: Laboratory diagnosis of typhoid fever. The approximate percentage of tests found positive during different stages of the disease (weeks 1–5) A. Widal agglutination. B. Feces culture. C. Blood culture

Third week

- Blood culture (yield 60 –70%).
- Widal test and clot culture
- Stool and urine culture.

Blood Culture Procedure

- Collect blood sample before starting antibiotics
- Select a site for collection
- Disinfect the area with Betadine starting from the center whirling concentrically outwards
- Wipe clean with spirit
- Wear sterile gloves and collect blood sample
- Amount to be collected – 5 ml for adult, 10 ml for children.
  - Transfer the sample to blood culture bottle containing brain heart infusion agar
  - Blood may be inoculated into bile broth which is an enrichment media for Salmonella
  - Casteneda's biphasic medium or liquid broth can also be used
- Transfer to lab immediately or if there is a delay incubate at 37 °C/Room temperature
- Collect at least 2 samples at an interval of 30 minutes from 2 different sites
- Never refrigerate the sample.

Incubate of inoculated BHIB at 37 °C for 7 days → Subculture on to solid culture media (blood agar, Mc Conkey agar).

Identification

- Gram's smear from the growth: Gram-negative
- Mc Conkey agar shows nonlactose fermenting
- Biochemical tests: oxidase negative
- S.typhi and S.paratyphi: produce H2S
- Final is by slide agglutination using specific antisera.

S. typhi	S. paratyphi A	S. paratyphi B
• Polyvalent O • O_9 antiserum (Group D antiserum). • D 'H' (flagellar antiserum)	• Polyvalent O • O_2 antiserum • A H antiserum	• Polyvalent O • O_4 antiserum • B H antiserum

3. Clotculture

- Lysed by streptokinase
- Advantage: Yield higher rate of isolation. Sample of serum also become available.

4. Feces culture

- During course of disease and in convalescence
- Occur in patient and carriers.

5. Serology

Widaltest

- For the measurement of H and O agglutinins for typhoid and paratyphoid bacilli
- Two types of tubes are generally used
  - Dreyer's tube: Narrow with conical bottom for H agglutination
  - Felix tube: Round bottom tube for O agglutination.

Procedure

- Equal volume of serial dilutions of serum H and O antigens are mixed in Dreyer's and felix agglutination tubes incubated water bath at 37 °C (Control tube are also set to check for auto agglutination)
- O agglutination: Disk like spreading in bottom
- H agglutination: Cotton wooly agglutination
- Significant titer: O > 100, H > 200
- Test become positive by 2nd week of fever.

Interpretation of Results

a. Titer depends on stage of disease, blood taken early may give a negative result
b. Demonstration of rise in titer of antibodies by 2 or more serum sample is more meaningful
c. Result of single sample should be interpreted with caution
d. Agglutinins may be present on account of prior disease, inapparent infection or immunization.
e. Bacterial suspension used as antigen should be free from fimbria.

Antigen detection

Advantages

- Early diagnosis
- Positive even after antibiotic therapy
- Simple bedside test.

Prophylaxis

- **General measures:** Improvement in sanitation. Provision of protected water supply
- **Vaccines:** TAB vaccine
  Live oral vaccine } Refer Vaccine section
  Vi vaccine

Treatment

- **Drug of choice:** Ciprofloxacin for ambulant patients.
  Ceftriaxone for toxic sick admitted patients.
- **Other drugs:** Chloramphenicol, Ampicillin, Cotrimoxazole, Azithromycin.

Multidrug Resistant Typhoid

- Resistant to Chloramphenicol ⟶ Treated by ampicillin, amoxicillin, Cotrimoxazole ⟶ become resistant to these drugs ⟶ Drug of choice Fluroquinolones, 3rd generation Cephalosporins.

15. Non-sporing Anaerobes

Examples
- Cocci: Vellionella (Gram–ve) Peptostreptococcus, peptococcus (Gram+ve)
- Bacilli: Nonsporing – Gram+ve– Eubacterium, Propioni bacterium Gram–ve– Bacteriodes, Fusobacterium
- Spirochetes: Treponema, Borellia
- Bacteroides fragilis is the most common isolate. They are non-sporing, non-motile, pleomorphic, capnophilic anaerobes. Commonly causes abscesses in brain and abdomen. Sensitive to metronidazole.

Common diseases
- CNS: Brain abscess – B. Fragilis, Peptostreptococcus
- ENT: Sinusitis, otitis – fusobacteria
- Mouth and Jaw: Gingivitis, Sinus of jaw – fusobacteria, spirochetes
- Respiratory: Bronchiectasis, empyema – B.fragilis, Fusobacteria
- Abdominal: Subphrenic and Hepatic abscess – B. Fragilis
- Genital infections: Puerperial sepsis – P. Melaningogenica, B. Fragilis
- Most infections are Polymicrobial.

Lab Diagnosis
- Specimen
  - anaerobes common inhabitant of skin and mucous surfaces
  - so mere presence not diagnostic
  - aspirations useful in lung abscess (but when aspirated in the syringes and penicillin bottles make sure that there is no air column)
- Transport and culture: Robertson's cooked meat medium
- Microscopy: Gram stained smear
- Culture – In Gaspak system or anaerobic jar, RCM.

Treatment
- Clindamycin and metronidazole most useful drugs
- Amoxicillin/Clavulanic acid combinations are also given.

16 Bordetella Pertussis

- Ovoid coccobacillus, capsulated, non-sporing
- Gram-negative with bipolar metachromatic granules
- Oxidase positive.

VIRULENCE FACTORS

- Agglutinogens
- Pertussis toxin (PT)
    - Lymphocytosis producing factor (LPF)
    - Histamine sensitizing factor (HSF)
    - Islet activating protien
- Filamentous hemagglutinin (Piracy of adhesion)
- Pertactin
- Others: Adenylate cyclase, heat labile toxin, tracheal cytotoxin.

Clinical Features
- Obligate human parasite
- Three stages
    a. Catarrhal: Clinical diagnosis difficult, stage of maximum infectivity
    b. Paroxysmal: Bouts of violent cough followed by inspiratory whoop through a narrow glottis
    c. Convalescent: Frequency of cough decrease.

Complications
- Pressure effects
- Respiratory: Bronchopneumonia, lung collapse
- Neurological: Convulsions, coma.

Epidemiology
- Highest in first year of life
- Spread: Fomites and droplets
- Maternal antibodies not protective.

Lab Diagnosis
- **Collection and transport of specimen**
  - Prenasal or nasopharyngeal swab (most important method)
  - Postnasal swab
  - Cough plate method
- **Microscopy**: Demonstration of bacili
- **Culture**: Glycerine potato blood agar of Bordet and Gengou
  Regan-Lowe medium

4. PCR
5. **Serology:** Not used
6. Other laboratory parameter: Leucocytosis (60–80% lymphocytosis)

Treatment
- Erythromycin (Drug of choice) and other newer Macrolides
- Chloramphenicol and cotrimoxazole is useful
- **Vaccine** (Refer vaccine section).

17 Haemophilus Influenzae

■ MAINLY CAUSE

- Meningitis: Bacteria spread from nasopharynx through bloodstream in children between 2 months and 3 years of age.
- Laryngoepiglottitis: A/C inflammation of epiglottis with obstructive laryngitis
- Pneumonia: Typically in infants and accompanied by empyema
- Suppurative lesions: Such as arthritis, carditis and pericarditis, otitis and cellulitis
- Bronchitis:

Pathogenicity

Disease caused may be categorized into 2 group:
1. Invasive Forms: Bacilli spread through blood protected from phagocytes by capsule
2. Noninvasive Forms: Bacteria spreads by local invasion by mucosal surface sinusitis, otitis, bronchitis

Lab Diagnosis

- Specimen: blood, CSF or sputum
- Microscopy: gram–ve showing pleomorphism
  - Nonmotile, non-sporing, capsulated
  - Cocco-bacilli: In sputum and young cultures Bacilli: in CSF and old cultures
- Direct Antigen Detection: Capsular polysaccharide antigen
- Culture
  - Requires factor V: NAD/NADP
    - Acts as hydrogen acceptor
    - Factor X: heme/porphyrin for cytochrome Enzymes for aerobic respiration
    - Chocolate Agar
    - Blood Agar with Staph. aureus shows satellitism
    - Nutrient Agar with factor X and V
    - Levinthals Medium
    - Fildes' Agar.

SATELLITISM

Staph. aureus streaked across a plate of blood agar with H.influenzae.
Over night incubates ↓
Large and well developed colonies of H.influenza near Staph. aureus

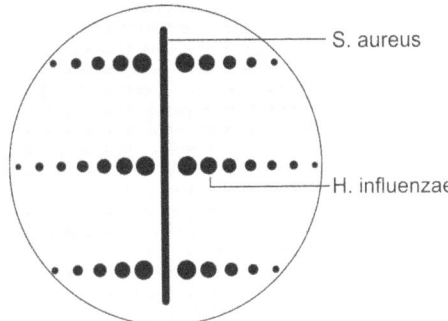

Fig. 17.1: H. influenzae on blood agar showing satellitism around S. aureus streaks

Treatment:
- Cefotaxime

Prevention:
- Hib vaccine (refer vaccines).

HAEMOPHILUS DUCREYI

Mainly produce chancroid/soft sore
Pathogenesis and clinical features:
- Venereal disease
- Tender, non-indurated irregular ulcers on the genitalia
- Regional lymph nodes enlarge and are painful.

Lab Diagnosis:
- Specimen: From lesion
- Microscopy: Gram–ve, arranged in groups
  Whorls-school of fish
  Parallel chains: Rail road track appearance
- Culture: Blood agar
  Chocolate agar enriched with isovitalex and fetal calf serum
- Animal inoculation
- Serology: Agglutination with antiserum.

Treatment
- Sulphonamides
- If resistant: Erythromycin, Cotrimoxazole, Ciproflocaxin/Ceftriaxone

HACEK Group Bacteria
Includes Haemophilus, Actinobacillus, Cardiobacterium, Eikenella, Kingella
Imp: Endocarditis.

18 Corynebacterium Diphtheria

- 'Gram-**positive** bacilli, non acid fast, irregularly stained segments and granules'
- Slender rod with tendency to form clubbing at one or both ends
- Contains Metachromatic granules which take up bluish purple color with Loeffler's methylene blue (Volutin or Babes Ernst granules)
- Albert's, Neiver's and Ponder's stain are also used
- Chinese letter or cuneiform arrangement of bacilli seen under microscopy

Morphology types : Gravis
  Intermedius
  Mitis

TOXIN

- Powerful exotoxin
- Standard strain (Park Williams 8 strain) used for toxin production
- **Factors:** Presence of corynephages (tox+) in bacteria (lysogenic conversion) Concentration of iron in medium
- **Mechanism of action:** inhibits protein synthesis
  - Fragment B helps in binding
  - Fragment A inhibits polypeptide chain elongation by EF2

Pathogenicity

- Incubation period: 3–4 days
- Sites: faucial, nasal, conjunctival, laryngeal, otitic, cutaneous, genital
- Classified on clinical basis into malignant, septic, hemmorhagic
- Complications: Asphyxia, a/c circulatory failure, postdiphtheritic paralysis, toxemia.

Lab Diagnosis

For confirmation and control measures
- Specimen: Swabs from throat
- Microscopy: Smear stained with special stains (vide supra) Bacilli with metochromatic granules
- Culture Isolation : Swabs inoculated on Loeffler's serum slope, Tellurite blood agar
- Demonstration of Toxicity: Virulence testing.

In Vivo

Subcutaneous test } on guinea pig
Intracutaneous test

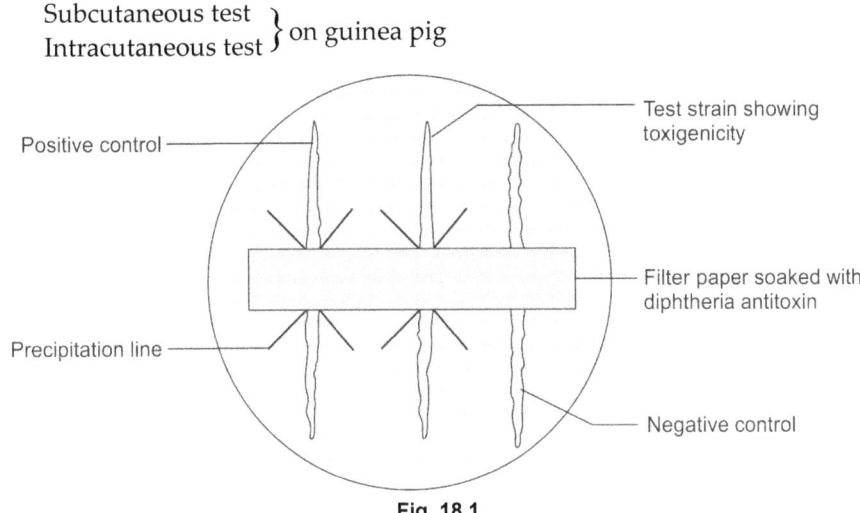

Fig. 18.1

In Vitro
Elek's gel precipitation test
- Rectangular filter paper strip with diphtheria antitoxin taken
- Placed on 20% normal horse serum agar
- Narrow streaks of test strains, positive and negative control are made at right angles to paper after agar sets
- Line of precipitation formed: Where toxin and antitoxin diffuse and meet
- Presence of arrow headline indicate toxigenic strain.

Tissue culture test
Prophylaxis
- DPT Vaccine
- Active, passive, combined
- Active: Formol toxoid (formalin)
    Adsorbed toxoid (aluminium phosphate/hydroxide)
    - dosage and vaccine - look vaccine section
- Passive: Emergency measure used in susceptible persons
    Subcutaneous administration [500–1000 IU] of ADS antitoxin
- Combined: First dose of adsorbed toxoid on one arm ADS on other arm.

Treatment
- Penicillin, Erythromycins are more active.

19 Pseudomonas

- Gram-negative motile non-sporing bacilli
- Saprophyte
- Obligate aerobe
- Oxidase +ve
- Causes opportunistic infections.

PSEUDOMONAS AERUGINOSA

Pigments are produced on culture
- Pyocyanin: Blue
- Pyoverdin: Green
- Pyorubin: Red
- Pyomelanin: Brown

Pathogenicity
- Exotoxin production-inhibit protein synthesis
- Nosocomial and community acquired infections
- Nosocomial ⟨ Localized / Generalized
- Community Acquired Suppurative otitis: (most common) Respiratory infections in cystic fibrosis patients
- Nosocomial: Wound infections
- Infections in burns patients

Eye infections
UTI in catheterized patients
Iatrogenic meningitis
Post-tracheostomy pulmonary infections
- Septicemia: Endocarditis, Ecthyma gangrenosum, Shangai fever.

Lab Diagnosis
- Identificaton of bacteria in clinical specimen
- Grows in ordinary media

- Selective media: Cetrimide agar
- Nutrient Agar: Pigment production
- Oxidase +ve reaction
- Species identification: Biochemical tests.

Treatment

- Ceftazidime, Cefaperazone, Cefepime
- Aminoglycosides
- Ciprofloxacin, piperacillin
- Resistant to most common disinfectants.

MELIOIDOSIS

- Caustive agent-Burkholderia pseudomallei
- Opportunistic infection.

Pathogenesis

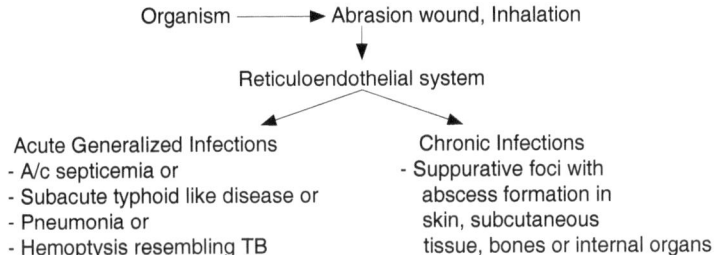

Predisposing Factors: Diabetes, Anemia, Renal diseases.

Lab diagnosis: Specimen depends upon type of infections.

Microscopy: Gram staining with methylene blue-Safety pin appearance.

Culture: Grows in ordinary media.

Serology: ELISA for IgG and IgM, IHA.

PCR

Treatment

- Ceftazidime is the DOC } long-term treatment due to reactivation or
- Cotrimoxazole, tetracycline } relapse
- Ceftazidime/Imipenem:
  2 wks + cotri/amoxyclav-6 wks

20 Brucella

- Gram-negative coccobacilli
- Noncapsulated, non-sporing, non-motile
- Strict aerobes
- Causative agent of brucellosis
- It is a Zoonotic infection
    - Br. melitensis-sleep
    - Br. abortins -cattle
    - Br. suis-pig

Brucella melitensis is the most pathogenic

Pathogenecity

Mode-Inhalation of wool, etc.
- Ingestion of animal products
- Contact-butchers, veterinary
- Lab contamination
- Reticuloendothelial system ← Bloodstream ← Lymph nodes

⎫ → Survive inside macrophages
⎬
⎭ → Lymphatic channels

Human Infection
- Latent
- **Acute** Brucellosis-fever, muscle pain, asthma, constipation, undulant fever, nervous system, osseous and ophthalmic Involvement
- **Chronic** low grade infections, sweating, lassitude, joint pain without pyrexia or minimal pyrexia

Lab Diagnosis
- Clinical diagnosis difficult
- A good history is useful
    - Specimen: Blood, Bone Marrow, lymph nodes, CSF, urine
    - Blood Culture: Most definitive method for diagnosis
    - Castaneda method: Incubation

Blood+Brucella broth ⟶ Subculture every 3–5 days
        $37\,°C, 5–10\ CO_2$
                                            ↓
                                       Growth
                            Kept for 6–8 weeks

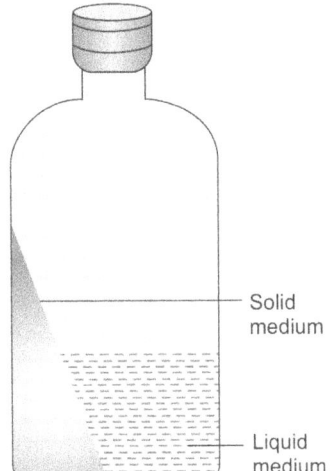

Fig. 20.1: Castaneda medium

Advantage: Both liquid and solid media available in same bottle reduce chances of contamination

Blood culture positive only in 30–50% cases

Newer BACTEC Methods-earlier isolation

- Serology.

Standard Agglutination Test

- Mainly identify IgM
- IgM antibodies declines as disease progress, IgG persists or rise in titer
- Positive in a/c infections and weakly positive or negative in c/c infections
- Demonstration of rise in titer-diagnostic
- Disadvantage-prozone phenomenon
  - ELISA: Both IgM and IgG separately
  - Rapid methods: Dipstick, Rose Bengal card test, milk ring test (for detection in animals)
  - Skin tests: Not useful in a/c brucellosis.

PROPHYLAXIS

- Checking of dairy animals
- Pasteurization of milk
- Vaccination in animals.

Treatment

- Doxycyclin + streptomycin ⟶ long-term treatment because it can survive
- Intracellularly
- Children: Cotrimoxazole with rifampicin or gentamicin
- Streptomycin: 2 weeks + doxycyclin: 45 days.

21. Mycobacterium Nonmycobacterium

- Gram-positive weakly acid fast (5% H_2SO_4) Bacilii
- Causative agent of leprosy
- Globi: Masses of bacilli bounded together by glia
- Seen inside histiocytes (tissue macrophages).

LEPROSY

- Chronic granulomatous disease, involving skin, peripheral nerves and nasal mucosa.

Madrid classification

- Lepromatous, Tuberculoid, Dimorphous, Indeterminate
- Lepromatous (Multibacillary disease)
- Large numbers of bacilli
- Cell mediated immunity deficient
- Involvement of nose, mouth, upper resp. tract (major), eyes, testes, reticuloendothelial system, kidneys and bones.

Ridley and Jopling Classification

- Tuberculoid (TT), Borderline tuberculoid (BT) and Borderline borderline (BB),
- Borderline lepromatous (BL), Lepromatous leprosy (LL).

Tuberculoid (paucibacillary)

- Scanty bacilli
- Adequate cell mediated immunity
- Neural involvement → deformity.

Lepra Reactions: Acute exacerbations in leprosy

Type 1 (Reversal reaction)

- Cell mediated immune reaction occurring spontaneously or during chemotherapy mostly in borderline leprosy
- Influx of lymphocytes into lesions
- Upgrading reaction: Shift to tuberculoid spectrum, (if treated)
- Downgrading reaction: Shift to lepromatous pattern in untreated or pregnant patients.

Type 2 (Erythema Nodosum Leprosum)
- Arthus type response seen in LL and BL types, few months after institution of chemotherapy
- Due to antigens released from dead lepra cell
- Tender subcutaneous nodules with fever, lymphadenopathy and arthralgia.

Lepromin Test
- To study immunity in leprosy patients
- Intradermal test
- Antigens used: 1. Mitsuda antigen (human) 2. Standard lepromin (lepromin A)
- Biphasic response

Early Reaction of Fernandez
— Erythema and induration develop in 24–48 hours.
— Persists for 3–5 days, little clinical significance.

Late Reaction of Mitsuda
— Starting in 1–2 weeks–peak in 4 weeks, subside in next weeks
— Indurated skin nodule becomes ulcerated
— Does not indicate pre-existing DTH, measure induced CMI.

Uses of lepromin test
- To classify leprosy
- To assess the prognosis and response to treatment
- To assess the resistance of individuals to leprosy
- To verify identity of candidate lepra bacilli.

Lab diagnosis
- Specimen: Nasal mucous membrane, skin, thickened nerve
- Culture: Not possible – only in foot pad of mice or nine banded armadillo
- Microscopy: AFB staining using 5% H_2SO_4
- Serology and molecular methods.

Treatment (refer pharmacology-WHO regimen)
- Dapsone, Clofazimine, Rifampicine, Ofloxacin, Minocycline.

Grading of smear
- 1–10 bacilli in 100 fields = 1+
- 1–10 bacilli in 10 fields = 2+
- 1–10 bacilli per field = 3+
- 10–100 bacilli per field = 4+
- 100–1000 bacilli per field = 5+
- More than 1000 bacilli, clumps = 6+

MYCOBACTERIUM TUBERCULOSIS

- Straight or slightly curved bacilli
- May occur in groups or singly
- It is an acid fast bacilli – stained by Ziehl – Neelsen staining
- Also gram-positive. (due to mycolic acid present in cell wall).

Pathogenicity

- It is a causative agent for Tuberculosis.

Mode of infection

- Direct inhalation of aerosolized bacilli in expectorated sputum.
- Often occurs by ingestion Through infected milk or rarely by inoculation.
  Bacilli inhaled (arrested by natural defenses) → Lungs (alveoli) → alveolar macrophages → Multiply in macrophages. CD4 + helper T cells → Cell Mediated Immunity → IFN-γ, IL-1 and IL-2, TNF-2 → Activate macrophages (epitheliod cells) → GRANULOMA formation (suppresses the progression).
- Tubercle (avascular granuloma)
  — Central zone of giant cells
  — Central caseation
  — Peripheral zone of lymphocyte and fibroblasts.
- Two types
  a. Exudative: In DTH response of host
  b. Productive: More protective immunity.

Factors affecting immunity

- Genetic susceptibility
- Age
- Immunocompetence
- Stress
- Nutrition

Classification Primary TB

- Initial infection by the bacilli in a host.
- In lower lobe or lower part of upper lobe in lungs they multiply to cause pneumonia (Ghon focus).
- Ghon focus + enlarged hilar lymph node – Ghon complex (3–8 weeks).
- After 2–6 months heals by calcification seen on X-ray (Ranke complex).

Post primary (secondary) TB

- Reactivation of latent infection or re-exposure
- In immunocompromised adults
- Affects mainly upper lobes and usually no lymph node involvement
- Lesion undergo necrosis and calcification
- Necrotic materials break out into airways leading to expectoration of infected bacilli
- Primary lesion may enlarge and cause miliary, meningeal or other forms of disseminated TB.

Lab Diagnosis

- Specimen
- Pulmonary TB: Sputum, bronchial washings (if sputum unavailable), Gastric lavage (children).
- Extrapulmonary TB:
  — Cold abscess: Aspiration/Biopsy (lymph node).
  — Renal TB: 3 early morning first voided sample on 3 consecutive days.
  — TB meningitis: CSF.
  — Others: Intestinal TB – biopsy intestine.
  — TB saplpingitis – biopsy fallopian tubes.
  — **Sample Collection: 2 early morning sample (RNTCP guidelines. One spot sample and another morning sample, collected in a wide mouth container after properly rinsing the mouth).**

I. Decontamination and concentration of specimens:

- Petroff's method
- NALC combined with 2% NaOH.

II. Microscopy

- AFB staining:
  a. ZN staining
  b. Kinyoun's method
  c. Gabet's method
- Fluorescent staining: Using Auramine O.

III. Culture

- Solid media: LJ medium – slower growth 37 °C– 4–8 weeks.
                Cream colored raised colonies. (Tarshi's, Loeffler's, Powlosky's media).
- Liquid media: Dubos medium (Middle brooke's medium) – Faster growth.
- Automated systems.

Identification of growth

- ZN staining
- Biochemical reactions
  a. Niacin test: Positive
  b. Catalase: Peroxidise test
     — Catalase: Weekly positive, Peroxidase: Positive
  c. Nitrate test: Positive
  d. Aryl sulphatase test: Negative.

IV. Antibiotic sensitivity testing

- Absolute concentration method
- Resistance ratio method
- Proportion method (more commonly used).

- MDR TB: Resistance to Rifampicin and INH with or without to any other 1st line drugs.
  XDR TB: MDR + Resistance to any quinolones and one injectable 2nd line drugs

No of bacilli	No of fields checked	Grading
No bacilli	100	-ve
0-9/100 field	100	Scanty, exact no of bacilli
10-99/100 field	100	1+
1-9/field	50	2+
>10	20	3+

V. Animal inoculation.
VI. Newer methods of diagnosis.
   - MODS
   - Automated Mycobacterial culture system – PCR, Line probe assay.

VII. Hypersensitivity Reactions

Mantoux test

   - Type IV hypersensitivity.
   - Only determine whether patient has been exposed to bacilli.
   - Can be due to infection or vaccination.
   - Intradermal injection of 0.1 ml PPD (5TU) flexor aspect with tuberculin syringe.
   - Examined after 48–72 hours.
   - Look for duration - > 10 mm - +ve
   - 5–10 mm – equivocal - < 5 mm - +ve
- Heaf test
- Tine test.

Interpretation of Mantoux

- Positive: Infection by bacilli.
- 4–6 weeks after immunization been positive.
- Negative: No contact of bacilli. False negative: Miliary TB Measles like infection
- Lympho reticular malignancies, Severe malnutrition
- Impaired immunity
- False positive: Atypical mycobacterial infection.

Prophylaxis: See Vaccine Section.

Treatment

- Antitubercular drugs are given.
- Bactericidal: Rifampicin(R), Isoniazid(H), Pyrazinamide (Z).
- Bacteriostatic: Ethambutol (E). (Regime: latest refer PARK).
- 2nd line drugs: PAS, amikacin, levofloxacin, rifabutin,
- Resistance: MDR-TB and XDR: TB strains.

- RNTCP
  - Launched in 1993.
  - Introduced DOTS
  - In MDR TB-DOTS plus.

NONTUBERCULOUS MYCOBACTERIUM

- Runyoun Classification
- Four groups based on pigment production.

Group	Nomenclature	Growth characteristics	Members
Group 1	Photochromogens	No pigment in dark. Become pigmented on exposure to light.	M.kansasii M.marinum
Group II	Scotochromogens	Pigmented in the dark light.	M.scrofulaceum M.gordonae
Group III	Non photochromogens	No pigment even on exposure to light.	M.avium M.intracellulare M.ulcerans M.xenopi
Group IV	Rapid growers	Growth within 7 days	M.fortuitum M.chalonae M.smegmatis

Skin Pathogens

Buruli ulcer
- Caused by M.ulcerans (only mycobacterium which produces toxin)
- Usual site: Leg or arms
- Mode of infection: Through minor injuries
- Indurated nodules appears, which break down forming indolent ulcers.

Mac Complex

- Mycobacterium aviumintra cellulare complex
- Pulmonary disease-especially in AIDS patients in developed countries.

Lab Diagnosis

- Smears from edge of ulcer show large clumps of bacilli-acid fast
- Later the bacilli disappears due to immunity.

SWIMMING POOL GRANULOMA

- Caused by M. Marinum
- Cause TB in fish and amphibians
- Mode of infection: Contaminated pools or fish tanks
- Lesion beginning as a papule and breaking down to form an indolent ulcer
- Usual site: Bony prominences-elbow, knee, ankle, nose, fingers or toes.

22 Spirochetes

- Gram-negative elongated, motile, flexible bacteria
- Presence of endoflagella is a feature
- Majority: Saprophytes, Others: Obligate parasites
- Aerobic/Anaerobic/Facultative.

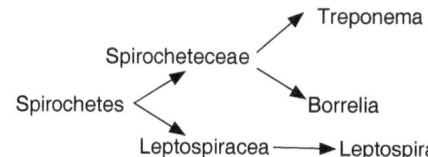

■ TREPONEMA

- Some are pathogenic. Others are commensals in mouth, intestine and genitals
- Causes following disease in human
- Veneral Syphilis – T. pallidum ⎫
- Endemic Syphilis – T. endemicum ⎬ Identical morphology and antigenic structure differ only in natural history and clinical features.
- Yaws – T. pertenue (body contact) ⎪
- Pinta – T. carateum ⎭

Treponema pallidum

- Actively motile spirochetes
- Not grows in culture media violates Koch's postulates
- Nichol's strain: Virulent strain:maintained by serial passage in rabbit testis
- Reiter's strain: Nonpathogenic strain.

Antigenic structure

- Nonspecific antigen (Reagin)
  - Induces reagin antibodies
  - Reacts with standard test for syphilis.
- Group antigen: Present in pathogenic and Non-pathogenic strains (Reiter's strain).
- Polysaccharide antigen: Positive in TP tests infected with pathogenic treponems.

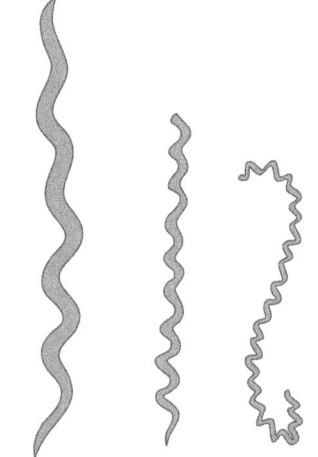

Borrelia   Treponema   Leptospira

Fig.22.1: Schematic representation of comparative morphology of different spirochetes

Mode of transmission
- Direct intimate contact (sexual or otherwise) with lesions containing spirochetes.
- Transplacental: Mother to fetus
- Blood transfusion during early syphilis
- Organ transplantation.

Clinical features

Primary Syphilis
- Chancre at site of entry
- Incubation period 10–90 days with average 21 days
- Painless, circumscribed, indurated, punched out lesions – Hard chancre (Hunterian chancre)
- Contain exudates rich in spirochetes
- Swollen, discrete, nontender, rubbery regional lymph nodes
- Multiple chancre – HIV infected/Immunodeficient individuals
- Sites of chancre:
    - Homosexual men: Anal canal, rectum, mouth or external genitalia
    - Heterosexual men: Penis.
    - Women: Cervix, labia.

Secondary Syphilis
- 1–3 months after the primary lesion heals
- Nonpruritic, roseolar/papular skin rashes characteristically involve palms and soles
- Mucous patches in oropharynx and condylomata at the mucocutaneous junction
- Fever, sore throat, fatigue, patchy hair loss and weight loss
- Most infectious during this stage — Ophthalmic, osseous and meningeal involvement.

Latent Syphilis
- After secondary lesion disappears
- Diagnosis only by serological test.

Tertiary Syphilis
- Cardiovascular lesions, chronic granulomata (gummata) and meningovascular manifestations.

Congenital Syphilis
- From mother to fetus transplacentally
- Occurs at any stage of pregnancy
- Higher chance in early syphilis
- Lesions develop after 4th month of gestation
- Adequate treatment before 4th month prevent congenital syphilis
- Untreated syphilis: Abortion and stillbirth
     Stigmata of syphilis and later healthy infants

- Diagnosis: Detection of IgM antibodies (FTA-ABS, TPHA, VDRL)
    Rise in titer of antibodies.

Lab Diagnosis of Syphilis

- Specimen: Exudates from lesion, Serum, CSF (neurosyphilis).
- Demonstation of organism
    - Light microscopy: Cannot take ordinary stains.
      Silver impregnation, Fontana, Negative staining,
    - Direct Fluorescent antibody test.
      Dark ground/Phase contrast microscopy: Wet film.
- Serological tests
    - Three classes of serological tests
    - STS – Standard test for syphilis (Reagin antibody test)
        For antibodies against cardiolipin antigen
    - Group antigen test
    - Specific antigen test

STS (nonspecific tests)

- Antibody reacting with cardiolipin: Reagin antibodies
- Cardiolipin used is extracted from beef heart
- VDRL/RPR: Slide flocculation test
- Wasserman: CFT.   Not done ⎫
- Kahn's test: Tube flocculation test ⎭ now

VDRL

- Venereal Disease Research Laboratory (VDRL) test
    - Slide flocculation type of Ag-Ab reaction
    - Simpler, more rapid and quantitative test
    - Inactivated serum (Serum heated at 56 °C for 30 minutes in water and cooled) is Mixed with 50 µl cardiolipin antigen on a special slide and rotated for 4 minutes
    - Forms visible clumps if serum contain regain antibodies
    - Read under low power microscope
    - For quantitative reporting: Reciprocal of highest dilution of serum is used.
    - Example: If highest dilution is 1/8, report is given as reactive 8 dilution Negative report as nonreactive
    - CSF can be also used for VDRL test, but plasma cannot used
    - Modification: RPR test – Rapid plasma reagin – charcoal coated cardiolipin antigen used. Automated RPR test: Large Scale testing
    - Automated VDRL ELISA test measuring IgM and IgG antibodies
    - ADV: Visual reading is more rapid (no microscope needed) No need of inactivation of serum.

Biological false positive reactions (BFP)

- Defined as positive reactions obtained in tests using cardiolipin antigen (i.e. STS) with negative results in specific treponemal tests, in the absence of past/present treponemal infection and not caused by lab errors.

- Due to presence of Cardiolipin antigen in Mammalian tissue
  - Major disadvantage of STS
- Acute BFP: Acute infections, injuries and inflammation.
  Lasts only for few weeks or months.
- Chronic BFP: SLE and collagen disease.
  Persists for longer than 6 months.
- Other conditions: Malaria, Leprosy, Relapsing fever, IMN, Hepatitis, Tropical eosinophilia.

Group specific tests

- RPCF (Reiter Protein Complement Fixation)

Specific tests

- TPI: Treponema Pallidum Immobilization: Gold standard in serology
- Fluorescent treponemal antibody (FTA): First test to become positive
- Treponema pallidum hemagglutination assay (TPHA)
- Enzyme immunoassay
- Prognostic indicator for treatment: VDRL (comes down after treatment). FTA antibodies of TPHA remains positive even after treatment.

Treatment

- Benzathine penicillin G – 2.4 million units single injection
- Ceftriaxone – Neurosyphilis.

LEPTOSPIRA

- Delicate spirochetes. (Umbrella handle appearance)
- Leptospira interrogans (Pathogens to human) cause leptospirosis
- Leptospira icterohemorrhagiae: Most pathogenic.

Pathogenesis

- Zoonotic disease
- Leptospires in water contaminated by the urine of carrier animals enter the body through cuts or abrasions on the skin or through mucosa of mouth, nose or conjunctiva
- Human-human transmission rare
- Damage to endothelial cells of small blood vessels
- Predisposing factors: Sewage work, flood, agricultural places.

Symptomatic Phase

- 7–12 days after infection
- Flu like symptoms: Sudden onset of headache. Muscle pain in back and calf. Fever with chills
- Conjunctival suffusion and skin rash seen in some.

Bacteremic Phase

- 7–8 days after symptomatic phase
- Spread to many organs and brain.

Symptoms
- Uveitis, meningitis, myocarditis.
- Hepatorenal dysfunction: Most fatal (WEIL'S Disease-L.icterohaemorrhagic)-(short note)
- Pulmonary hemorrhagic syndrome.

Immune Phase
- Appearance of antibiotics and disappearance of leptospires from blood
- Show signs of recovery.

Biphasic
- Fever, headache and meningism returns
  - Bleeding.
  - Jaundice: liver enzyme moderately elevated
  - Renal impairment.

Pulmonary Manifestation
- ARDS - death.

Lab diagnosis
- Specimen: Blood, urine.
- Microscopy
  - Dark ground microscopy (1st week): Will remain in blood only for 1 week then goes to kidney
  - Urine microscopy: 2nd week of disease.
  - Culture: EMJH media.
- Serology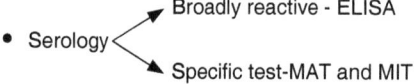
  - Broadly reactive - ELISA
  - Specific test-MAT and MIT

Detection of specific antibody
- Positive on 6th day
- Detection delayed in prior antibody therapy
- 4 fold rise in titer of antibodies in convalescent and disease stage.
- Microscopic agglutination test
  - Gold standard
  - Genus specific antibody detected
  - Tells infecting serogroup
  - Cross reaction between difference serovars, agglutination, absorption tests may sometimes necessary.

Clinically
- ELISA for IgM antibody
- Molecular methods: PCR.

Prophylaxis

- Rodent control, disinfection of water and wearing protective clothing and vaccination in high-risk agricultural workers.

Treatment

- Benzyl penicillin: DOC.
- Doxycyclin: Prophylaxis.

LYME DISEASE

- Also known as Lyme Borreliosis.
- A new spirochetal disease, resembles juvenile rheumatoid arthritis
- Causative organism: Borrelia burgdorferi
- Vector: Ixodid ticks.

Epidemiology

- Widespread in USA
- Also in other parts of world.

PATHOGENESIS AND CLINICAL FEATURES:

- Mode of infection: Regurgitation of gut contents during bite from Ixodid ticks
- Occurs in 3 stages
    1. Localized infection – expanding annular skin lesion (erythema migrans
    2. Disseminated infection – fever, headache, myalgia, arthralgia
    3. Persistent infection – chronic arthritis, polyneuropathy, acrodermatitis.

Lab Diagnosis

- Specimen: From skin lesions, ticks, CSF, blood of patients
- Isolation: By culture in modified Kelley's medium
    - Culture too slow, so less importance in diagnosis
- Serology:
    - ELISA and IF: Identification
    - Immunoblotting: Confirmation.

Treatment

- Doxycycline, amoxicillin and cefuroxime are useful.

23 Mycoplasma

MYCOPLASMA/PLEUROPNEUMONIA LIKE ORGANISMS

Morphology

- Gram –ve, stains with Giemsa
- Devoid of cell wall, can pass through filters
- No fined size or shape
- Seen as granules and filaments
- Multiplication by binary fission asynchronously: Chains of beads produced
- Some shows bullous enlargement by means of which organisms attach themselves to suitable host
- Shows hemadsorption, e.g. M.pneumoniae, M.hominis, Ureaplasma urealyticum.

ATYPICAL PNEUMONIA

- Caused by M. pneumoniae
- Typically it is tracheobronchitis
- Mode of transmission: droplets of nasopharyngeal secretion
- Characterized by fever, headache, malaise and sore throat, paroxysmal cough with blood stinged sputum
- Paucity of respiratory sign on physical examination, Radiographically: Consolidation affecting lower lobe, patchy, starting at hilum and fanning out to periphery.

Lab Diagnosis

- **Sample collection:** Throat swab and respiratory secretion
- **Transport media:** Mycoplasma media
- **Isolation:** Complex media PPLO broth (biphasic medium).

Identification of Growth:

- Fried egg appearance
- Acid production in medium
- Beta hemolysis and agglutinates guinea pig erythrocytes
- Tetrazolium reduction test: Reduction of colorless tetrazolium into red color.
- **Microscopy:** Stained by Diene's method: block is cut out from Methylene blue and azur red added.

- Molecular methods
- Serology
- Specific tests
  - Immunofluorescence
  - Hemagglutination inhibitor
  - Growth inhibition test
  - Complement fixation test
- Nonspecific tests.

a. Streptococcus MG test

- Serial dilution of patient's unheated serum and heat killed suspension of streptococcus
  Overnight incubation ↓
- Agglutination (Significant titer: > 20.)

b. Cold agglutination test (heterophileagg.)

- Based on appearance of microglobulin against human group O cells
- Serial dilution of patient's serum + 0.2% washed erythrocytes.
  Incubation at 4 degree Celsius ↓
      Clumping observed
  37 degree Celsius ↓
      Clumping dissociates.

Treatment

- Tetracyclin and Doxycyclin.

UREAPLASMA UREALYTICUM

- Second most common cause of non gonococcal urethritis
- Via sexual contact
- Cause – urethritis, Proctitis, Balanoposthitis and Reiter's syndrome in male. Acute salpingitis, PID, cervicitis and vaginitis in women
- Associated with infertility, abortion, postpartum fever, chorioamnionitis and LBW of infants.

24 Miscellaneous

ACTINOMYCETES

- Gram-positive, non-motile, break-up to coccoid and bacillary elements
- Causes Actinomycosis: Chronic granulomatous infection
- Facultative anaerobes:
- Common – A.israelli.

Pathogenicity

- Normal flora of intestine, mouth and vagina
- Invasion occurs in trauma/foreign bodies or poor oral hygiene.

Clinical Features

- Indurated swellings, suppuration and discharge of sulfur granules are bacteria colonies
- Come out as multiple sinuses
- Four main clinical forms: Cervicofacial most common.
  - Thoracic
  - Abdominal
  - Pelvic

Lab Diagnosis

- Specimen: Pus or tissue, sputum
- Examination of granules: White or yellowish
- Microscopy: Demonstrate actinomycetes and granules. Bacteria as Sun-ray appearance
- Isolation and culture: Thioglycollate medium or BHIB. Spidery colonies on solid media.

Treatment

- Prolonged treatment with penicillin or tetracycline.
- Supplemented by surgery if necessary.

LISTERIA MONOCYTOGENES

- Non-sporing Gram-positive bacillus
- Aerobic or microphilic and peritrichous flagella
- Motility occurs only at 25 °C
- Tumbling motility.

Epidemiology

- Widely distributed in nature.
- Human infection caused by serovar 1/2a or 1/2b and 4b.
- Route of infection – contact with infected animal, ingestion of animal products milk, meat, egg etc.

Pathogenicity and Clinical Features

- Intracellular organism which survive inside PMNL'S
- In pregnant women: Causes abortion/stillbirth.
- In neonates: **Meningitis** or sepsis.
- In Immunocompromised: Meningoencephalitis
- Listeriolysin O: Virulence factor.
- May be present as pharyngitis, urethritis, pneumonia, IMN like syndrome.

Lab Diagnosis

- Specimen:
    - Cervical or vaginal secretions.
    - Meconium or cord blood.
    - Blood and CSF.
- Demonstration of bacilli: Incubate under 5% CO_2 on blood agar.
- Isolation: Cold enrichment method.
- Serology: Antibody to listeriolycin O.

Treatment

- Ampicillin, Cotrimoxazole, Gentamicin.

Prevention

- Proper preparation of food by washing vegetables.
- Pasteurization of milk and through cooking.

ACINETOBACTER BAUMANNI

- Strictly aerobic, Gram-negative coccobacillary rods
- Oxidase negative
- Nonfermenters
- Classified under genomo species of Acinetobacter.

Pathogenicity and Clinical Features

- Opportunistic pathogens
- Health care associated infections (Ventilator associated pneumonia, meningitis, bacteremia)
- Multidrug resistant causes greater therapeutic challenge.

Treatment

- Following standard precautions is best strategy.

HELICOBACTER PYLORI

- Gram-negative spiral bacilli
- Motile: Lophotrichous flagella
- Production of urease.

Mechanism of Transmission

- Not clear
- Likely to be feco-oral or oral–oral route.

Pathogenicity

- Does not invade but colonizes the gastric mucosa
- Commonest site – gastric antrum
- Bacterial protease, toxins or ammonia released by urease
- Activity on autoimmune responses to gastric antigens also contribute.

Clinical Features

- Mild acute gastritis or asymptomatic
- Peptic ulcer disease
- Chronic atrophic gastritis – later stages
- Acts as risk factor of MALTomas, adenocarcinoma of stomach

Lab Diagnosis

Invasive tests

- Specimen: Endoscopic biopsy of gastric mucosa
- Piece of material put in urease medium: Positive result
- Microscopy of biopsy sections: Gram staining and silver staining.

Noninvasive Tests

- Serology by ELISA
- Urease breath test.

Treatment

Triple drug regimen
- Lansoprazole 30 mg
- Amoxicillin 1 g   } bd 14 days
- Clarithromycin 500 mg

LEGIONELLA PNEUMOPHILA

- Gram-negative noncapsulated bacilli, coccobacillary in clinical material
- Causes legionnaires pneumonia
- Polar flagella.

Epidemiology
- Human infection by inhalation of aerosols (Air coolers, AC, etc.)
- No carrier state or human to human transmission
- Risk factors: smoking, alcohol, advanced age, immunodeficiency.

Pathogenicity
- Aerosols ⟶ alveoli ⟶ Multiply inside monocytes and macrophages
- Cellular immunity is responsible for recovery.

Clinical Features
- Two distinct patterns:
  - Legionaire's disease
    - Fever, nonproductive cough, dyspnea
    - Untreated: End in pneumonia
    - Diarrhea and encephalopathy common.
  - Pontiac disease
    - Mild, nonfatal, 'influenza like illness'.
    - Outbreaks with high attack rates occur.

Lab Diagnosis
- Specimen: Sputum, bronchial aspirate and lung biopsy
- Selective media: BCYE (Buffered Chewed Yeast Extract)
- Demonstration: By fluorescent antibody test
- Serology: Latex agglutination or ELISA. Identify legionella antigens in urine.

Treatment
- Newer macrolides, ciprofloxacin
- Rifampicin is used in severe cases.

25 Rickettsiaceae

- Small, gram-negative bacilli
- They are virus like and are obligate intracellular parasite
- Three genera: 1. Rickettsia. 2. Orientia 3. Ehrlichia

Genus Rickettsia
- Consist of causative agents of 2 groups of diseases
- Typhus fever caused by Ricketsiaprowazeki and R.typhi
- Spotted fever caused by R.typhi.

TYPHUS FEVER

- Caused by R.prowazeki
- This group of disease consists of epidemic typhus, endemic typhus and recrudescent typhus.

Morphology
- Gram-vecoccobacilli
- Nonmotile noncapsulated
- Stains with Giemsa and casteneda ⟶ bluish purple.

Epidemic Typhus
- R.prowazeki
- Vector: Headlice
- Get infection on feeding rickettsial patient
- Mode of transmission: **Feces** ⟶ through abrasion produced by scratching.
  Aerosols of dried feces through inhalation.
- Multiply locally ⟶ enters blood ⟶ localized to endothelium ⟶ cell enlarged, degenerates and thrombi formation ⟶ partial or complete occlusion
- A/C febrile illness characterized by septicemia, Maculopapular lesion sparing face, sole and palm.

Recrudescent Typhus
- Brill Zinsser disease
- After recovery rickettsia remain latent in lymph node which get activated.

Endemic Typhus
- R.typhi
- Reservoir – rat
- Vector – Xenopsyllacheopis (rat flea)
- Mode of infection – rubbing, aerosol contamination.

Scrub Typhus
- Also known as chigger –borne typhus
- Causative agent: Orientiats utsugamushi
- Vector: trombiculid mite.

Pathogenesis
- Mite island (focussed to an area) → man get infection by bite of mite larvae (chiggers) → feeds on warm blood
- Reservoir – rodents and birds
- Four factors essential for establishment of infection 1. O.tsutsugamushi. 2. Chiggers 3. Rat 4. Secondary form of vegetations
- Causes Eschar at site of lesion, Maculopapular rash, Lymphadenopathy, fever, headache and conjunctival injection.

Genus Ehrlichia
- Infect WBCs
- In cytoplasm of infected phagocytic cells → grow within phagosome → mulberry like cluster (morula).
- Causes: → Glandular fever: lymphoid hyperplasia and atypical lymphocytosis
    → Human monocytic Ehrlichcosis: associated with leucopenia, thrombocytopenia and elevated liver enzymes
    → Human granulocytic Ehrlichiosis.

LAB DIAGNOSIS OF RICKETTSIAL DISEASES

- **Specimen:** Blood, tissue for culture, serum for serology, skin biopsy
- **Direct Microscopy:**
    Light microscopy: Aggregates of rickettsial particle in cytoplasm Giemsa stain— purple bluish in clusters
    Machiavello's stain: Red colored inclusion
    Skin biopsy: Immunofluorescence, immunohistochemical and immune enzymes. Morula can see in case of Ehrlichiosis
- **Culture:** Yolk sac of embryonated eggs.
    - Male guinea pig or mice Cell and tissue culture

- Animal inoculation
- **Neil Mooser reaction or tunica reaction shown by R.typhi**
  - Intraperitoneal inoculation → scrotum enlarges → testis cannot push back because of inflammatory adhesions between layers of testis
- **Serological tests:**
  Weil Felix reaction: (short note)
  - Heterophile agglutination test
  - Used for serodiagnosis of typhus fever
  - Based on sharing of a common antigen between typhus ricketssiae and some strains of proteus bacilli
  - Sera tested for agglutinins to O antigen of proteus strain OX19, OX2, OX K
  - Antibodies appears rapidly during course of disease and reach peak by 2nd week and declines rapidly
  - Usually done as tube agglutination test
  - Proteus is isolated from urine of patient.
  - Advantage: Simple and useful for diagnosis of ricketssial disease
  - Disadvantage: Not used for early diagnosis

Disease	Agglutination	Pattern	With
	OX 19	OX 2	OX K
Epidemic typhus	+++	+	-
Brill-Zinsser disease	Usually –ve or weakly +ve		
Endemic typhus	+++	±	-
Tickborne spotted Fever	++	++	-
Scrub typhus	-	-	+++

- **Molecular diagnosis– by PCR**

Treatment
- Tetracyclin and Ciprofloxacin.

Q FEVER

- Caused by Coxiella species
- Gram-vecoccobacilli
- Nonmotile, noncapsulated
- Intracellular parasite of monocyte, macrophage cell.

Pathogenesis
- It is a zoonosis.
- Humans get infection through handling of wools, meat or other animal products contaminated with bacterium.
- Entry: abraded skin/mucosa, lungs/intestinal tract
- Causes: A/C systemic infection-causing influenza like illness C/C Q fever – Endocarditis, meningitis, hepatitis.

Lab Diagnosis
1. Specimen: Blood for culture and microscopy
    - Serum for serology
    - Vegetation from heart
2. **Microscopy**: Machiavello's stain – red inclusion
3. **Culture:** Yolksac, tissue
4. **Serology:** Micrsoagglutination, CFT, ELISA, IFT
5. **Molecular methods:** By PCR.

26 Chlamydiae

- Obligate intracellular parasites
- Tropism: Squamous epithelial cells, macrophages

Have features of both virus and bacteria.

Viral Features

- Pass through filters
- Failure to grow in cell-free media
- No peptidoglycan cell walls.

Bacterial Features

- Posses both DNA and RNA
- Have rigid cell walls
- Multiply by binary fission
- Susceptible to antibiotic
- Do not have eclipse phase following cellular infection.

MORPHOLOGY

- **Elementary body (EB)**
  - Extracellular infective form
  - Spherical particle
  - Rigid trilaminar cell wall and nucleoid
- **Reticulate body (RB)**
  - Intracellular growing and republica form
  - Fragile and pliable cell wall
- **Inclusion bodies:**
  - Developing chlamydial microcolony within the host cell
  - C.trachomatis ⟶ compact inclusions with glycogen matrix (HP bodies)
  - C.psittaci ⟶ diffuse vacuolated inclusion without glycogen matrix (Levinthal Cole Lillys bodies).

Growth Cycle

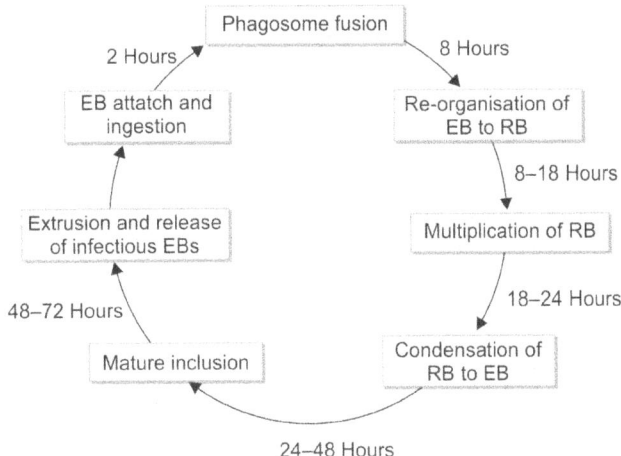

Antigens

- LPS: genus specific (complement fixation test)
- Envelop Protein Antigen: species specific (ELISA)
- Major outer membrane protein: Intra species typing (micro –IF), Biovars (TRIC, LGV) and serotypes.

Species	Disease	Serotype	
C. trachomatis	Endemic trachoma	A, B, Ba, C	
" "	Inclusion conjunctivitis, Genital chlamydia Infant pneumonia	D, E, F, G, H, I, J, K	Tric agents
" "	Lypmho granuloma venerum	L1, L2, L3 → LGV	
C. psittaci	Psittacosis	Many serotypes	
C. pneumonia	A/C resp disease	Only one serotype	

Pathogenesis

- Ocular infection: Trachoma, inclusion conjunctivitis, ophthalmia neonatorum
- Genital infection
- Respiratory infection.

TRACHOMA

- Chronic keratoconjunctivitis
- Major cause of blindness: Follicular hypertrophy, pappilary hyperplasia, pannus formation, cicatrization.

Genital chlamydiasis

- Non-Gonococcal urethritis
- Reiter's syndrome
- Fitz-hugh-Curtiz syndrome.

Lymphogranulomavenerum-climate/tropical bubo/poradenitis
- Scarring and lymphatic blockage – elephantiasis of vulva.

Psittacosis – parrot's man (occupational) – Bird fancier's disease
- Mild influenza like syndrome
- Pneumonia
- Septicemia
- Meningoencephalitis.

C. pneumonia
- Taiwan acute respiratory strain
- Group specific antigen
- Exclusively human
- Associated with atherosclerosis: Coronary, carotid, cerebral.

Lab Diagnosis
- Demonstration of inclusion bodies and elementary bodies
- Direct detection of antigens
- Demonstration of antibodies
- Isolation of chlamydia
- Skin test-Frie's intradermal test for LGV.
    a. **Specimen:**
    — Conjunctival scrapings-trachoma
    — Urine
    b. **Microscopy:**
    - Giemsa, Castenada, Macchiavello stains
    - Trachoma inclusion body: Halberstaedter-Prowazek bodies (HP bodies)
    c. **Direct detection:** Immunofluorescence: More sensitive and specific
    - ELISA
    - DNA probes PCR
    d. **Serology:** Antibody detection by complement fixation test
    e. **Isolation:** Animal Inoculation, yolk-sac chick embryo
    f. **Tissue culture:** He La Cells.

Treatment
- Trachoma: Erythromycin and Tetracyclin
- LGV: Sulfonamides and Tetracyclin
- C.pneumonia: Clarithromycin and azithromycin.

27 General Properties of Viruses

MORPHOLOGY

Size
- Smaller than bacteria
- Extracellular infectious virus particle—virions

Structure and shape Capsid
- Nucleic acid surrounded by protein coat
- Capsid made of capsomeres
- Has protective function
- Three kinds of symmetry: Icosahedral, helical, complex

Envelope
- Host cell derived
- Made of lipoprotein
- Protein spikes projecting on surface of envelope—Peplomers, e.g. hemagglutinin, neuraminidase
- Confers chemical, antigenic and biological properties.

Viral Hemagglutination
- A large number of viruses agglutinate erythrocytes from different species
- Due to presence of hemagglutinin spikes on surface of virus, e.g. Influenza
- Influenza carries enzyme neuraminidase which act on receptor and destroys it, therefore Neuraminidase called Receptor destroying enzyme (RDE) and the process is termed as ELUTION.
- Hemagglutination test can be carried out in test tubes
- Red cells are added to serial dilution of viral suspension

  ↓

  Settle at bottom
- Highest dilution producing hemagglutination—Hemagglutination titer
- They are inhibited by antibody
- In case of myxovirus, elution occurs due to presence of neuraminidase
- Virus which have eluted from red cells are capable of agglutinating fresh red cells
- But red cells that have been act on by virus are not susceptible to agglutination by same strains.

Cultivation of Viruses

a. Animal Inoculation
- Suckling mice (arboviruses, coxsackie), guinea pig, rabbits are used
- Growth of virus indicated by death, disease or visible lesions
- Routes: Intracerebral, sc, intraperitoneal
- Disadvantages: Immunity may interfere with viral growth and that animals Harbor latent viruses.

b. Embryonated Eggs
- Provides different sites for cultivation
- Chorio allantoic membrane: Produces visible lesions (pocks), e.g. Variola/Vaccinia
- Allantoic cavity: Influenza and some paramyxoviruses
- Amniotic sac: Primary isolation of Influenza virus
- Yolk sac: Chlamydiae and Rickettsiae.

c. Tissue Culture

Organ culture	Explant culture	Cell culture
By using small bits of organs, e.g. Coronaviruses in tracheal ring	Fragments of mixed tissue, e.g. Adenoviruses in adenoid tissue	Tissue dissociated into component cells ↓ Cells washed and counted ↓ Suspended in growth medium Antibiotics added to prevent contamination

Cell Culture

Primary Cell Culture	Diploid cell strains	Continuous cell lines
Capable of limited growth Cannot maintain serial cultures Use: Isolation and vaccine production, e.g. monkey kidney, human embryonic kidney, human amnion, chick embryo	Cell type capable of retaining original diploid chromosome after serial subcultivations Use: Vaccine production, e.g. human fibroblasts	Cells capable of continuous serial cultivation indefinitely Derived from human cancers HeLa, Hep-2, KB

■ DETECTION OF VIRUS GROWTH IN CELL CULTURES

a. Cytopathic effect
- Morphological changes in cultured cells in which viruses grow
- Such viruses are termed as Cytopathogenic viruses, e.g.
    - Measles: Syncitium
    - Herpes: Discrete focal degeneration
    - Adenovirus: Bunch of grapes like granular clumps
    - SV 40: Cytoplasmic vacuolation.

b. Metabolic inhibition
c. Hemadsorption

d. Interference
e. Immunofluorescence.

Classification of Viruses

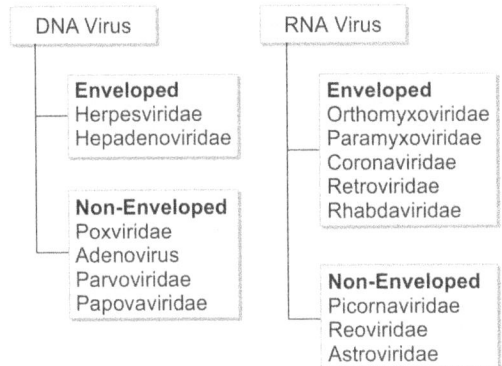

VIRUS HOST INTERACTIONS

Inclusion Bodies

Definition
- Structures with distinct size, shape, location and staining properties that can be demonstrated in virus infected cells
- Seen under light microscope
- Most characteristic histologic feature in virus infected cells.

Based on
- **Staining properties**
  - Acidophilic: Seen as pink structures with Giemsa or Leishman stain
  - Basophilic: Adenovirus have such inclusions
- **Site**
  - Cytoplasm: Poxviruses
  - Nucleus: Herpesviruses
  - Both: Measles virus
- **Composition**
  - Crystalline aggregates of virions or viral antigens seen at site of viral synthesis
  - Some represent degenerative changes produced by viruses
- **Intracytoplasmic Inclusions**
  - Cowdry type A: Herpesvirus, yellow fever virus
  - Cowdry type B: Adenovirus, Poliovirus
- **Diagnostic Importance**
  - Negri bodies: Rabies
  - Guarnieri bodies: Vaccinia
  - Bollinger bodies: Fowlpox
  - Molluscum bodies: Molluscum contagiosum.

INTERFERON

Definition
- Family of host coded proteins produced by cells on induction by viral or nonviral inducers
- Interferons act on other cells and same species rendering them refractory to viral infection
- Interferon ⟶ Cells ⟶ Traslation inhibiting peptide (TIP) ⟶ Block viral protein synthesis
- TIP [Protein kinase, Oligonucleotide synthetase, RNAase]
- Interferons are species specific but not virus specific
- Viruses vary in their susceptibility to interferon and RNA viruses are better inducers than DNA viruses
- Potent inducers: Toga viruses, Vesicular stomatitis virus, Sendai virus and NDV
- Efficient inducers: ds RNA and some synthetic polymers (poly 1: C)
- Interferon production increases by increasing temperature 40 °C
- Inhibited by steroids and increased O_2 tension
- Production is much quicker than antibody response.

TYPES: Based on antigenicity, cell of origin and other properties
- **IFN-α (leucocyte interferon):**
  - Produced by leucocytes
  - Nonglycosylated protein
- **IFN-β (fibroblast interferon):**
  - Produced by fibroblasts and epithelial cells
  - Glycoprotein
- **IFN-γ (immune interferon):**
- Produced by T-lymphocytes
- Immunomodulatory and antiproliferative functions
- Has separate cell receptor
- Acid labile.

Clinical Uses
- Ideal candidate for use in prophylaxis and treatment of viral infections
- Species specificity drawback is overcome by producing it from buffy coat leucocytes from blood banks
- Local application: URTI, Herpetic keratitis, genital warts (high doses)
- Limited success against Generalized herpes infection in immunocompramised, Hep B and C.

Biological Effects
- Antiviral effects
- Antimicrobial effects
- Cellular effects
- Immunoregulatory effects.

28 Bacteriophage

- Virus that infects bacterium
- Has role in transduction, phage conversion and recombinant DNA technology.

Morphology

- Tadpole shaped with head and tail
- Head: Hexagonal shape
- Contains packed core of nucleic acid covered by capsid
- Tail: Consists of hollow core and terminal base plate, which has prongs, tail fibers or both.

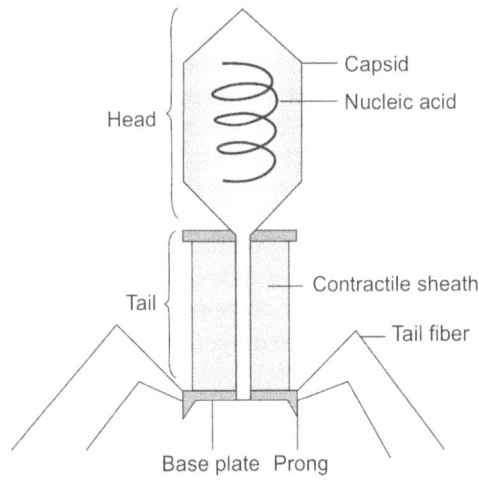

Fig. 28.1: Morphology of bacteriophage

Life Cycle

Two types of life cycle
1. Lytic Cycle: Intracellular multiplication of phage lead to cell lysis
2. Lysogenic Cycle: Cause no harm to cell, phage DNA becomes integrated with bacterial genome.

1. Lytic Cycle:

- Phases
    - Penetration
    - Synthesis of phage compounds

- Assembly
- Mature
- Release of progeny

Adsorption:
- Occurs when bacteria collides with phage
- Attaches by its tail
- Takes place in presence of complimentary chemical groups on receptor site on bacteria and base plate of phage
- Receptor site maybe in different site of cell wall
- Bacterial protoplast cannot adsorb phage
- Transfection: Infection of bacterium by naked phage

Penetration:
- Basal plate and tail fiber strongly hold against cell
- Pierce by hollow core
- Contractile sheath provides energy
- DNA inserted through hollow core
- Head and tail remains attached to host – Ghost
- **Lysis from without:** Bacteria get infected by large number of phage

  ↓

  Multiple holes were made on the cell

  ↓

  Bacterial lysis occurs without multiplication of phage

Synthesis:
- Early protein: First product to be synthesized for building of complex molecules
- Late protein: Protein subunits of phage head and tail
- During this period bacterial molecules synthesis stops.

Maturation:
- Phage DNA, head protein and tail protein are synthesized separately
- DNA is condensed and incorporated into head: Packaging
- Maturation: Assembly of phage compound into infective phage particles.

Release:
- During replication of the phage, bacterial cell get swollen and weakened

  ↓

  Phage enzyme act on the weakened cell wall

  ↓

  Bacterial lysis
- Eclipse phase: Interval between entry of nucleic acid into bacterial cell and appearance of first infectious intracellular phage particle
- Latent period: Interval b/w infection of bacterial cell and first release of infectious phage particle
- Rise period: Period during which no. of infectious phage released rises
- Burst size: Average yield of progeny phages

  Infected bacterial cell

2. Lysogenic Cycle

- Phage DNA integrated into bacterial DNA
- Incorporated phage nucleic acid: Prophage
- Bacterium carrying prophage: Lysogenic bacterium
- Phage confers certain properties on lysogenic bacterium: Lysogenic conversion or phage conversion
- Spontaneous induction of prophage

Sometimes prophage get excised
↓
Initiates lytic replicate
↓
Daughter phage particles released
↓
Infect other bacteria
↓
Render them lysogenic

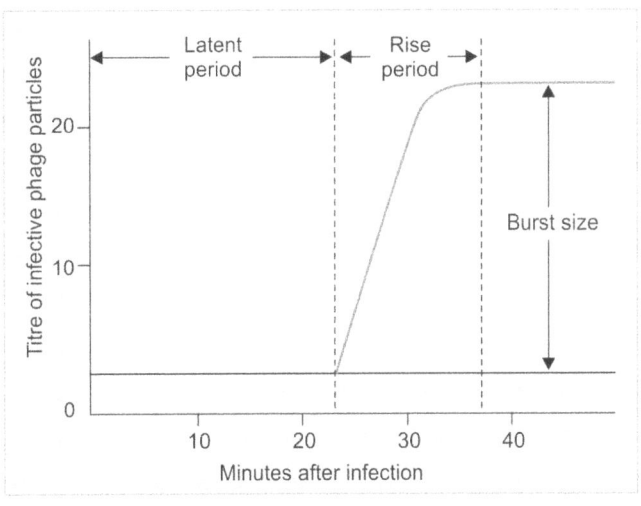

Fig. 28.2: One-step growth curve of bacteriophage

Significance

- Phage Assay: Phage applied to lawn culture incubation
  ↓
  Zone of lysis called Plaques
- Phage Typing: → Group specific
  → Species specific
  → Subspecies specific

29 Herpesviruses

- Enveloped dsDNA viruses
- Latent infections: Characteristic
- Icosahedral: Double stranded DNA
- Intranuclear Cowdry type A (Lipschutz) inclusion bodies.

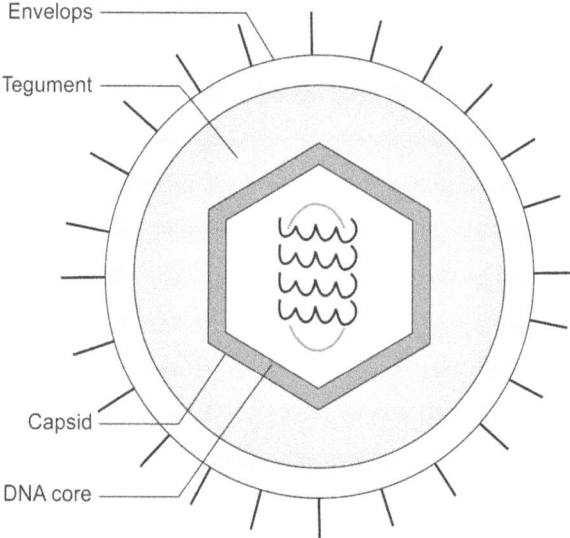

Fig. 29.1: Herpes simplex virus

Three Subfamilies

Alpha herpes viruses
- Short replicative cycle
- Latent infections in sensory ganglia, e.g. Herpes Simplex, Varicella Zoster.

Betaherpes viruses
- Replicates slowly
- Narrow host range
- Enlargement of infected cell (Fibroblast) – cytomegaly
- Latent infections in salivary and other glands, e.g. CMV.

Gammaherpesviruses

- Narrow host range
- Latent infections in lymphoid tissue.
  Example Epstein – Barr virus.

HERPES SIMPLEX – HHV 1 AND 2

- Natural host: Only humans
- HHV1: Oral lesions
- HHV2: Veneral disease

	HSV-1	HSV-2
Site	In and around mouth	Genital herpes
Mode of spread	Direct contact/droplet	Sexual
Latency	Trigeminal	Sacral

Pathogenesis

- Sources of infection: Saliva, skin lesion, resp. secretions, asymptomatic carrier also
- Virus $\xrightarrow{\text{Skin/mucous membrane}}$ Local multiplication and cell–cell spread $\longrightarrow$ Cutaneous nerve fiber $\xrightarrow{\text{Intra-axonally}}$ Ganglia $\xrightarrow{\text{Centrifugal migration}}$ Skin and mucosa lesions
  HSV1: Trigeminal
  HSV2: Sacral
- Primary infection will be systemic
- Recurrent infection-localized
- Periodic reactivation from ganglia
- Antibodies do not prevent recurrence
- Lesions: Thin walled umbilicated vesicles $\xrightarrow{\text{Breaks down}}$ Superficial ulcer $\longrightarrow$ Heals
- General rule HSV1: Above the waist
- Not absolute HSV2: Below the waist, (but rule is not absolute).

Clinical Features

Cutaneous

- (Face, cheek, around mouth, buttocks: Babies)
- Fever blister or herpes febrilis
- Herpetic whitlow: In doctors, nurses, dentists
- Eczema herpeticum: Infants resemble Kaposi's varicelli form eruption.

Mucosal

- Buccal mucosa most common site
- Gingivostomatitis and pharyngitis.

Herpetic keratitis

- HSV1
- Accompanied by conjunctivitis

- Dendritic ulcer in cornea
- Scarring and corneal blindness
- Choreoretinitis uncommon but serious.

Encephalitis

Most common cause of sporadic viral encephalitis
- HSV meningitis: Self-limiting
- Sacral autonomic dysfunction, transverse myelitis, GBS.

Visceral

- Esophagitis
- Tracheobronchitis
- Pneumonitis.

Genital

- STD
- Oncogenic potential: Cervical carcinoma
- Neonatal
- Congenital malformations: Rare
- Infection during birth: HSV2
- Postnatal infections: HSV1

Lab Diagnosis

Specimen: Vesicle fluid, skin swabs, saliva, corneal scrapings, CSF.

Microscopy
- **Tzanck smear**: From lesions – stain with 1% toluidine blue solution
  Multinucleated giant cells with faceted nuclei
  Homogenously stained ground glass chromatin
- Giemsa stain: Cowdry type A inclusion bodies
- Electron microscope
- Fluorescent antibody technique.

Virus isolation

- Human embryonic kidney
- Human amnion, human diploid fibroblast.

Serology

- ELISA
- CFT
- HSV1 and 2 differentiated by PCR and molecular methods.

Chemotherapy

- Acyclovir,
- Valacyclovir, Famcyclovir, Fencyclovir.

HHV-3 VARICELLA ZOSTER VIRUS

- Chickenpox: Primary infection in nonimmune individual.
- Herpes zoster: Reactivation of latent virus when immunity falls.

CHICKENPOX (VARICELLA)

Mostly in childhood, can occur in any age.

Pathogenecity and Clinical Features

- Source of infection: Chickenpox or herpes zoster patient
- Route of entry: Respiratory tract or conjunctiva
- Incubation period: 7 to 23 days
- Patient infectious 2 days before and 5 days after the onset of rash
- Rashes of various stages (pleomorphic rash)
- Macule, papule, vesicle, pustule, and scab
- 'Dew drops on rose petal' appearance of rashes
- Centripetal distribution of rashes (trunk 1st, limbs spared)
- Adults: Bullous and hemorrhagic lesions.

Complications

- Varicella pneumonia: Especially adults: most serious complications
- Myocarditis, nephritis, acute cerebellar ataxia, meningitis
- Reye's syndrome: h/o administration of salicylates.

Chickenpox in Pregnancy

- Maternal varicella in 1st half of pregnancy
    - Asymptomatic fetal infection or
    - Fetal varicella syndrome
- Maternal varicella near delivery
    - Congenital or neonatal varicella

Mother's rash > 1 week of delivery ⟶ Virus + antibodies —Transplacental route→ No clinical disease to child

Mother's rash < 1 week of delivery ⟶ Only virus —Transplacental route→ Neonatal varicella

Lab Diagnosis

- Usually clinical
- **Microscopy:** Tzanck smear
    Multi nucleated giant cell and cowdry type A inclusion bodies
- **Virus isolation**
- **Serology:** ELISA and PCR.

Prophylaxis

- Varicella vaccine
  - Live vaccine, c/i in pregnancy, subcutaneously given
  - 1st dose 1–12 years
  - 2nd dose > 12 years
- Varicella immunoglobulin.

Treatment

Acyclovir

■ HERPES ZOSTER (SHINGLES, ZONA)

- Old age: Usually > 50 years
- Most common segment T3 – L2 and ophthalmic branch of trigeminal nerve
- Reactivation of virus in sensory ganglia when immunity waned.

Complications

- LMN palsy, ramsay hunt, herpes zoster opthalmicus

■ HHV 4-EPSTIEN–BARR VIRUS

Causes

- Infectious mononucleosis: Kissing disease
- EBV associated malignancies
  - Burkitt's lymphoma
  - Lymphomas in immunodeficient patients: Hodgkin's, non-Hodgkin's, etc.
  - Nasopharyngeal carcinoma.

Pathogenicity

Source of infection: Saliva of infected persons via intimate close contact.

Virus ⟶ Pharyngeal cell ⟶ Local multiplication
↓
Infected B lymphocytes with CD 21 receptors ⟵ Bloodstream
↙   ↘
Latent inside lymphocytes   Cell death
↓   ↓
Polyclonal activation   Release of mature virions
↓
Immunoglobulins

IMN (Glandular Fever) – Short Note

- Acute self-limited illness charecterized by fever, sore throat, lymphadenopathy and presence of abnormal lymphocytes in peripheral blood.
- Seen in young adults.

Clinical Features
- Maculopapular rash and subclinical hepatitis
- Hematological, neurological, cardiac and pulmonary complications and splenic rupture

Lab Diagnosis
- Blood examination: Peripheral smear.
    Atypical lymphocytes: Kidney shaped nuclei and deeply basophilic vacuolated cytoplasm.
- Serology
    - Paul-Bunnell Test: Standard diagnostic test (Hetrophile Ab agglutination test against sheep RBC's)
    - Immunofluorescence and ELISA
    - Ab to EB nuclear antigen and VCA (viral capsid antigen)
    - PCR.

Treatment
Acyclovir.

HHV 5 – CYTOMEGALOVIRUS

- Salivary gland viruses
- Largest of herpes virus
- One of the most common organism causing intrauterine infection
- Largest of the herpesviruses enlargement of infected cells (cytomegaly) and owl's eye appearance
- Spread: Saliva, Sexual, Blood transfusion, Vertical and organ transplantation.

Clinical Features
- Causes intrauterine infection
- Congenital infections: Cytomegalic inclusion disease of newborn
- Infection in infants
- Infection in children (post-transfusion mononucleosis)
- Transplant recipients: Diffuse interstitial pneumonia between 1 to 6 months of transplantation

Lab Diagnosis
- Specimen: Urine, Saliva, Semen, Cervical secretions
- Isolation: Human fibroblast detection of inclusion bodies in cells-owl's eye
- Serology
    - Now ELISA
    - PCR: CMV DNA

Prevention and Treatment
- In organ transplants immunodefficient persons and premature infants
- Screening of blood and organ donors
- No vaccine available
- Ganciclovir: Treatment
    HHV-6: Roseolainfantum/Exanthema subitum/6th disease.
    HHV-8: Associated with Kaposi's sarcoma.

30 Orthomyxoviruses

INFLUENZA VIRUS

Causes influenza

Influenza: Acute infectious disease of respiratory tract which occurs in sporadic, epidemic and pandemic forms

Morphology

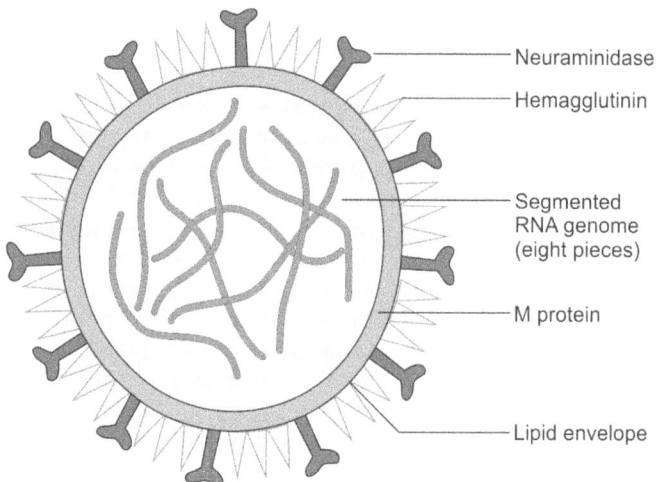

Fig. 30.1: Influenza virus

Antigens: ⟶ Internal antigen (RNP antigen) ⟶ M protein antigen
⟶ Surface antigen (V antigen) ⟶ Hemagglutinin and Neuraminidase

- **Hemagglutinin:**
  - Enables virus to adsorb to mucoprotein receptors on RBC and respiratory epithelial cells
  - Four distinct human subtypes.
- **Hemagglutination:**
  - Important characteristic of influenza virus
  - Virus links together adjacent RBCs forming hemagglutination.
- **Neuraminidase:**
  - Destroys cell receptors by hydrolytic cleavage
  - Strain specific antigen and exhibits variation
  - Nine subtypes are seen (N1–N9).

Antigenic Variation (S.note)
- Unique features of Influenza viruses: Important in epidemiology of disease
- Highest in influenza type A whereas less in type B and not seen in type C
- Only surface antigen undergo variations.

Two Types

1. Antigenic Drift
- Gradual sequential change in antigenic structure occurring regularly at frequent intervals
- New antigens are still related to previous
- Thus react with antisera to produces virus strains
- Accounts for periodic epidemics.

2. Antigenic Shift
- Abrupt, drastic, discontinuous variation resulting in novel strain
- Unrelated to previous virus strain
- Causes major epidemic or pandemic
- Changes involved are too extensive to be accounted for by mutation.

Pathogenicity

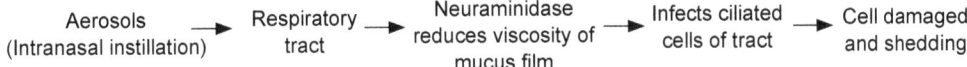

Aerosols (Intranasal instillation) → Respiratory tract → Neuraminidase reduces viscosity of mucus film → Infects ciliated cells of tract → Cell damaged and shedding

Clinical Features
- Spectrum: Mild coryza → fulminant pneumonia
- Abrupt onset with fever, headache and generalised myalgia
- In type B: Abdominal pain and vomiting and Reye's syndrome
- Complications: Cardiac – CCF CNS – encephalitis.

Lab Diagnosis
- **Demonstration** of virus antigen in nasopharyngeal cells by immunofluorescence
- **Isolation of virus**
  - Sample: Throat gargling using broth saline.
- **Specimen Treated** with antibiotics to destroy bacteria
  - Isolation maybe in egg or monkey kidney cells
  - Amniotic/allantoic fluids are tested for hemagglutination

  Type A virus: Only guinea pig cells

  Type B virus: Both guinea pig and fowl cells

  Type C virus: Only fowl cells.
- Serology: CFT and hemagglutination inhibition test
- Hemagglutination inhibition
  - Detection and quantification of antibody to virus
  - Advantage: Serological diagnosis of influenza

- Disadvantage: The presence of certain non-specific substances that can inhibit hemagglutination
- Procedure: Serum diluted in HA plates ⟶ virus suspension added ⟶ fowl RBC added.
- Highest dilution that inhibits HA ⟶ HI titer.
• PCR based diagnosis.

Immunoprophylaxis
- Used when pandemic threatened by new virus
- Two types
  - Inactivated vaccines, Subunit vaccines,
  - Recombinant vaccines Live attenuated (cold adapted) vaccines.

Treatment and Chemoprophylaxis
- Amantadine and Rimantidine are useful
- Newer drugs: Zanamivir and Oseltamivir.

31. Paramyxoviruses

Orthomyxoviridae	Paramyxoviridae
Segmented 8 pieces of RNA	Single linear RNA
Genetic reassortment common	No genetic reassortment
Antigenic variability	Antigenic stability
H and N on different spikes	H and N on same spike

PARAMYXOVIRIDAE

- Mumps virus
- Measles virus
- Respiratory syncitial virus
- Parainfluenza virus

Mumps

- Caused by Rubulavirus

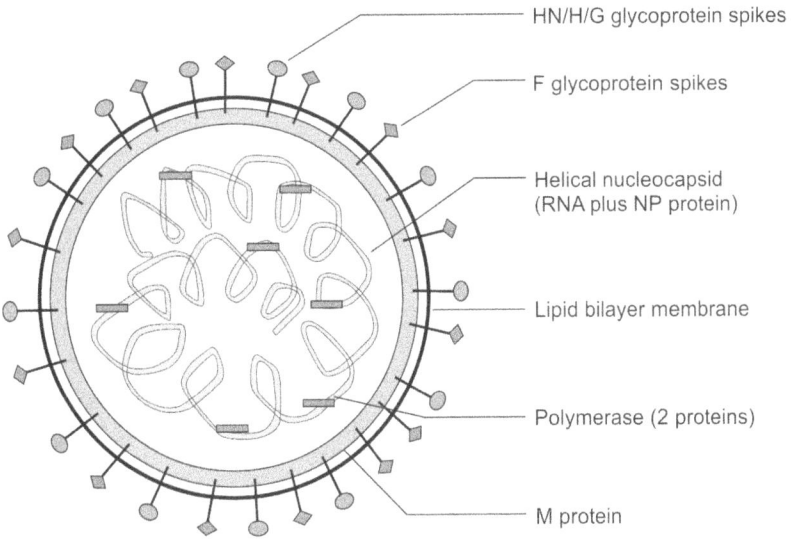

Fig. 31.1: Mumps virus

Rubulavirus
- Single antigenic type
- Hemagglutinim spike H
- Neuraminidase spike N
- F protein.

Pathogenesis
- Mode of spread
  - Direct contact
  - Inhalation
  - Fomites contaminated with saliva/conjunctiva
- Incubation period – 12 to 25 days
- Peak infectivity – 1 or 2 days before parotitis
- Replicates in upper respiratory tract and cervical nodes
- Disseminated through blood to various organs.

Clinical Features
- Fever, malaise, nonsuppurative parotid swelling
- Tenderness over parotid area
- Skin over the gland not warm or erythematous.

Complications
- Epididymo-orchitis – 10% patients
- Especially postpubertal males
- Testis: Swollen and painful
- Bilateral: Sterility, low sperm count
- Aseptic meningitis: Leads to deafness
- Less common: Arthritis, oophoritis, nephritis, pancreatitis, thyroiditis, myocarditis.

Lab Diagnosis
- Usually clinical
  - Specimens
  - Saliva
    - Urine
    - CSF
- **Viral isolation**
  - Monkey kidney culture
  - HeLa or Human amnion
  - Hemabsorption: Identified by hemadsorption inhibition using special antiserum
    Syncitia formation } Cytopathic effects
    Acidophilic cytoplasmic inclusions
- **Direct antigen** detection: IFA
- **Serology**: IgM, ELISA, Hemagglutination inhibition
- **Reverse transcriptase** PCR (Rt PCR).

Prophylaxis

- Vaccine
  - Live attenuated vaccine
  - Jeryl–Lynn strain
  - Single subcutaneous injection
  - MMR vaccine
  - Protection for 3 years

Measles

Caused by Morbillivirus

Morbillivirus

- Hemagglutinin spike H
- Neuraminidase spike N
- F protein.

Pathogenesis

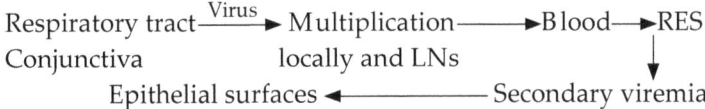

Respiratory tract —Virus→ Multiplication locally and LNs → Blood → RES → Secondary viremia → Epithelial surfaces

Conjunctiva

Clinical Features

- Incubation period 9 to 11 days
- Prodromal features: Malaise, fever, conjunctival injection, cough, nasal discharge
- Koplik's spots:
  - Bluish white ulcers seen in buccal mucosa
  - Pathognomic
  - Contain giant cells, cytoplasmic and intranuclear inclusion and virion complexes
  - Indication of local viral replication.
- Maculopapular rash
- Croup bronchitis
- Pneumonia, otitis media: 2° to bacterial infections
- Meningoencephalitis: Most serious
- Subacute Sclerosing Panencephelitis [SSPE]
- Diarrhea
- Suppression of delayed type hypersensitivity
- Spontaneous abortion or premature delivery: Pregnant woman.

Lab Diagnosis

- Clinically
- **Specimen:** Nasal secretions, throat swab, conjunctiva, blood.

1. Direct microscopy
   - Giemsa staining
   - Presence of multinucleated giant cells —Warthin–Finkeldey cells.

2. Virus isolation
- From nose, throat, conjunctiva
- Monkey kidney cell and primary human cell
- Cytopathic effects: Syncytia formation.

3. Serology
- Hemagglutination inhibition
- Complement fixation test

4. IFA–Ag detection
5. RT–PCR.

Prophylaxis
- Live vaccine
- Edmondson Zagreb strain-9 months
- Single, s/c
- Or MMR.

Parainfluenza Virus
- Four types: 1, 2, 3, 4
- Causes respiratory infections in children
- Most important is croup.

Lab Diagnosis
1. Specimen: Throat and nasal swab
2. Virus isolation: Hemadsorption on Monkey kidney culture
3. Serology
4. PCR.

■ RESPIRATORY SYNCYTIAL VIRUS

- Most important cause of respiratory tract infection in young infants
- No hemagglutinin activity
- **Clinical features**: Bronchiolitis, pneumonia and otitis media in young children
- No vaccines available.

Lab Diagnosis
- **Specimen:** Nasopharyngeal Swabs/Washings
- Inoculated into cell cultures: Forms Multinucleated Syncytia
- Serology: ELISA PCR

Treatment: Supportive

32 Arbovirus

- O'Nyongvirus
- Semliki family: Togaviridae
- Genus: Alphavirus
- All of them are mosquito-borne
- For examples, Encephalitis virus, Chikungunya virus, D'nyong forest virus, Sindbis virus.

CHIKUNGUNYA

- Caused by Chikungunya virus
- ssRNA virus.

Pathogenesis

- Insect bite ⟶ Multiply in RES ⟶ Blood (viremia) ⟶ Organ
- Virus enters via bite of Aedis aegypti.

Clinical Features

- Biphasic pattern of fever (remission after 1–6 days)
- Lymphadenopathy
- Crippling joint pain
- Maculopapular rash.

Lab Diagnosis

- **Specimen:** Blood
  Serum for serology
- **Isolation:** Animal inoculation using suckling mouse
- **Detection by:** Hemagglutination inhibition
  Complement fixation
  Gel precipitation
  ELISA
- **Molecular:** Rt PCR

```
                    Family: Flaviviridae
                   /                    \
          Mosquito-borne              Tick-borne
          Encephalitis virus          Encephalitis virus
          Yellow fever                Hemorrhagic virus
          Dengue fever
```

JAPANESE ENCEPHALITIS

- Most serious
- Characterized by onset of fever, headache, and vomiting (1–6 days)
  ↓
- Nuchal rigidity, convulsions, altered sensorium, coma
- Vector: Culex tritaenorhyncs
          Culex vishui
- Blood: Neutrophil leucocytosis
- CSF: Pleocytosis, increased glucose and protein levels.

Lab Diagnosis
Same as that for Chikungunya

CONTROL MEASURES

- Mosquito control
- Vaccines:
  - Formalin inactivated mouse brain vaccine using Nakayama strain 2 doses at two weeks interval
 Booster 6 months later
  - Live attenuated vaccine
  - JE strain SA 14-4-2
  - 2 doses, 1 year apart.

YELLOW FEVER

- Caused by yellow fever virus
- 2 cycles

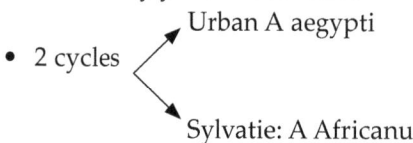

Clinical Features
Sudden onset of fever, headache, nausea 7 vomiting.

Lab Diagnosis

- Same
- Control: 17 D Vaccine by passing Asibi strain.

DENGUE FEVER

- Caused by dengue virus
- Also known as break bone disease
- 'Clinically similar to Chikungunya and **O'Nyong'**
- Virus is of 4 types: DEN 1, DEN 2, DEN 3 and DEN 4
- Immunity is type specific, so person has four episodes of dengue
- Vector: Aedes aegpti.

Clinical Features

- Sudden onset of fever, headache, vomiting, retrobulbar pain, conjunctival congestion
- Pain in back and limbs
- Lymphadenopathy, Maculopapular rash
- Severe: Dengue hemorrhagic fever.
- Dengue shock syndrome

Lab Diagnosis

- Same as above.

KYASANUR FOREST DISEASE

- Reported in Kyasanur forest in Karnataka
- Vector: Haemophilus sphingera
- Antigenically similar to Russian spring summer encephalitis.

Clinical Features

- Fever, headache, conjunctivitis, myalgia, Hemorrhage into skin, mucosa, and viscera.

Lab Diagnosis

Same as that of other Arbovirus.

33 Rabies Virus

- Bullet shaped, enveloped, ssRNA viruses.
- Belong to Lyssa virus genera of Rhabdoviridae
- Causes Rabies or Hydrophobia

Morphology

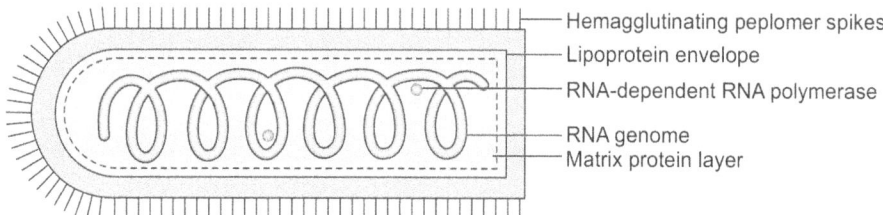

Fig. 33.1: Rabies virus

Antigenic Properties

- Glycoprotein spikes
  - Helps in binding
  - Stimulates cytotoxic T-cell immunity
  - Used in vaccine preparation.
- Nucleoprotein
  - Induces complement fixing antigen
  - Group specific antigen
  - Used in diagnostic immunoflouresence tests.

Host Range

- Street virus: Virus isolated from human/animal infection, negri bodies are seen in brain of such animals
- Fixed virus: Produced by serial intracerebral passages in rabbits, no negri bodies are formed.

Pathogenesis

Bite from rabid animal [exposure]
        Multiplies in new host [IP–90 days]
                ↓

Virus spreads to CNS and reaches brain [1st symptom]
↓
Pain and symptoms at site of inoculation [prodromal stage]
↓
Cerebral dysfunction, anxiety, confusion, agitation [1st neurological sign]
Delirium. Hallucination. Hydrophobia, aerophobia, photopobia [a/c neurologic phase
↓
Coma
↓
Death

Clinical Stages: As said above

Lab Diagnosis

- **Specimen:** Corneal smears, skin biopsy, saliva antemortem, brain postmortem.
- **Direct Microscopy:**

Antemortem: Rabies virus antigen demonstrated by immunofluorescence.
Postmortem: Negri bodies demonstrated in brain.

Isolation

- Animal inoculation: Intracerebral inoculation in mice from brain, saliva, CSF and urine: Isolated
- Tissue culture: Rapid and sensitive method
- Antibody demonstration: Seen in CSF in high titer
- Molecular method: Rabies virus RNA detected by recombinant PCR.

Demonstration of Negri Bodies

- Negri bodies seen in brain more in hippocampus and cerebellum
- Seller's technique:
  - Impression smear of brain stained by basic fuchsin and methylene blue in methanol
  - Seen as intracytoplasmic, purplish, round/oval structures with basophilic inner granules
  - If negative stained by Giemsa or Mann's method
- Demonstration of rabies viral antigen by immunofluorescence.

Prophylaxis

Vaccine section.

34 Hepatitis Virus

TYPE A HEPATITIS

- Caused by hepatitis A virus
- Single stranded RNA virus, Nonenveloped
- Mode of transmission : feco-oral route
- Infection by ingestion of contaminated food, water or milk.

Pathogenesis

- Entry through food ⟶ Multiply within intestine ⟶ Reaches liver via blood
- Shed on feces during late incubation period
- No transplacental infection.

Clinical Features

- Two phases:
    1. Prodromal/preicteric ⟶ Fever, malaise, nausea, vomiting, liver tenderness
    2. Icteric phase.
- Viremia seen during late incubation period and prodromal stage.

Lab Diagnosis

- **Specimen:** Feces or serum
- **Demonstration:** By immune electron microscopy
- **Serology:** Detection of antibody
    - IgM during late IP ⟶ Peaks ⟶ Disappears often
      (2–3 weeks) (3–4 months)
    - IgG persists much longer
    - IgM demonstration denotes recent infection.

Prophylaxis

- Good hygiene, sanitation
- Immunization:
  Active: Formalin inactivated alum conjugated vaccine containing HAV grown in human diploid cell culture.
  2 doses IM
  Passive: Pooled gamma immunoglobulin, given IM.

HEPATITIS B VIRUS [HBV]

- Cause more severe form of hepatitis
- dsDNA virus, enveloped.

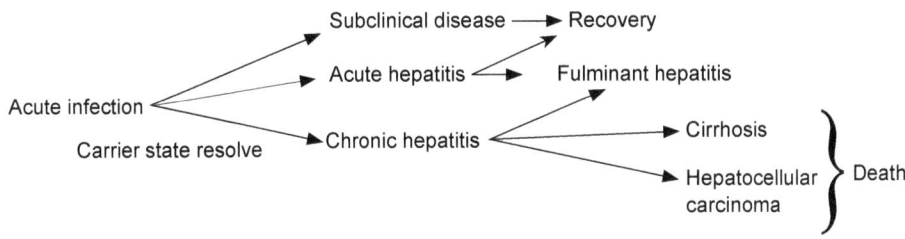

Fever, malaise, nausea, vomiting, liver tenderness, jaundice.

Antigenic Diversity

- HBsAg: exhibits antigenic diversity
- HBcAg:
   Virus $\xrightarrow{\text{mild detergents}}$ core/nucleocapsid expressed $\longrightarrow$ HBcAg
- HBeAg: Soluble non-particulate nucleocapsid protein secreted into fluid
- Viral genome:
  - dsDNA
  - Positive strand $\longrightarrow$ incomplete, has DNA polymerase

  DNA dependant DNA polymerase   RNA dependant reverse transcriptase
- Contains 4 overlapping genes
  - S gene → surface antigen
  - C gene
  - P gene
  - X gene

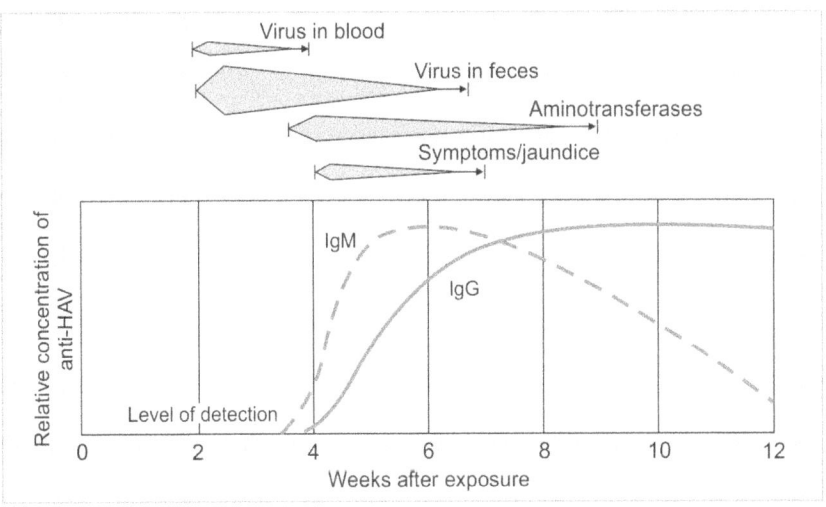

Fig. 34.1: Immunologic and biologic events associated with human infection with hepatitis A virus

Epidemiology

Carriers
- Super carriers–high HBsAg, HBV DNA, HBeAg
- Simple carriers–low HBsAg

Transmission

- Parental transmission
  - More risk if mother contains HBcAg
  - Infection acquired by contact of maternal blood with skin or mucosa of the fetus
- Sexual transmission
- Occupational risk.

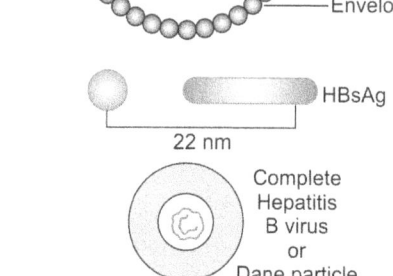

Fig. 34.2: Structure of hepatitis B. virus

Lab Diagnosis

By demonstration of viral markers.

HBsAg

- 1st marker to appear in blood after infection
- Before evaluation of transaminases and onset of illness
- Remains in blood throughout icteric phase/symptoms
- Falls from 2nd month onwards and lasts for 6 months
- Followed by anti-HBs antibody.

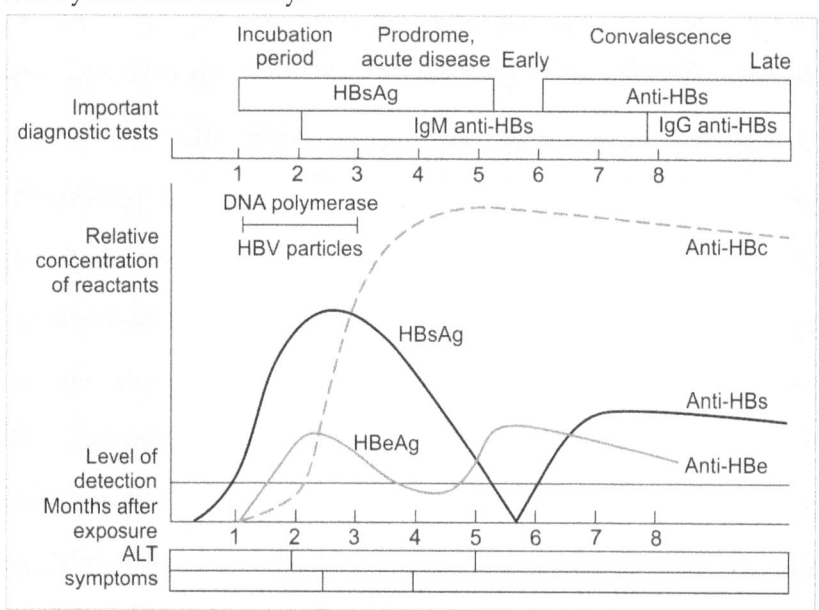

Fig.34.3: Clinical and serologic events occurring in a patient with acute hepatitis B virus infection

HBcAg
- Not found in blood
- Present in hepatocytes
- Anti-HBcAg in blood –
    - IgM: Recent infection
    - IgG: Remote infection
- 1 week after appearance of HBsAg
- 1st antibody to appear
- Provide lifelong protection
- If only HBcAg is present without other markers ⟶ prior infection

HBeAg
- In blood
- Presence indicates high infectivity and replication
- Its fall coincides with that of transaminases.

Diagnosis
- Detection of HBsAg
- If IgM HBcAg + HBsAg ⟶ Denotes recent infection
- IgG antibody ⟶ Remote infection
- Absence of HBeAg ⟶ Less infective
- Anti-HBs without any other serological markers

Molecular Diagnosis
- DNA hybridization
- PCR.

IMMUNIZATION

Passive
- Hepatitis B immunoglobulin
- IM, 300–500 IU

Active
- Genetically engineered subunit vaccine
- Content: Nonglucosylated HBsAg particles with alum adjuvant
- Dose 1 ml for adults
    - 0.5 ml for children
- Route: IM
- Site: Deltoid.
Anterolateral aspect of mid thigh in children
- Schedule: 0, 1, 6 months

Hepatitis C Virus

Contact with blood and blood products, vertical transmission.

Clinical Features
- Acute illness is mild
- Rarely develop jaundice
- Progress to acute hepatitis, cirrhosis, and hepatocellular carcinoma.

Lab Diagnosis
- Standard method: Antibody detection by ELISA
- Molecular diagnosis: PCR.

Prophylaxis
General prophylaxis, no specific immunizing agents available.

Treatment
Interferon alpha.

35 Slow Virus Diseases

FEATURES OF SLOW VIRUS INFECTION

- Ranging from months to years
- Course of illness months to years
- Predilection for involvement of CNS
- Genetic predisposition
- Invariable fatal termination
- Absence of immune response/an immune response that does not arrest the disease.

Classified into 3 Groups
Group A

- Consists of slowly progressive infection of sheep
- Causative agent: Nononcogenic retrovirus called lentivirus
- Visna: Demyelinating disease of the sheep
- Medi: Slow progressive fatal hemorrhagic pneumonia of sheep.

Group B (Prion Disease) * IMP

- Infectious agent is protenaceous, devoid of DNA and RNA – PRIONs
- The subacute spongi form viral encephalitis are c/c progressive degenerative disease of CNS

Pathogenesis

Proliferation of an abnormal prion protein PrpSC
↓
Accumulation of CNS as amyloid plaques
↓
Disrupts architecture and functioning of brain

Pathology

- Vaculotion in dendritic and axonal process
- Astroglial hypertrophy and proliferation
- Spongiform degeneration in grey matter.

Prion Disease of Animals Scrapie
- Mink encephalopathy
- Bovine spongiform encephalopathy (mad cow disease)

Human Prion Diseases
1. Creutzfeldt-Jakob disease–sporadic (common)
   - Inherited
   - Iatrogenic
- Occurs after corneal transplantation and ingestion of growth hormones
- Characterized by progressive incoordination and dementia.
2. KURU
   - Lead to cerebellar ataxia and tremors
   - Infection introduced trough cannibalizm
3. GSS: Gerstmann–Straussler–Scheinker syndrome
4. Fatal familial insomnia.

Group-C
- Subacute sclerosing pan encephalitis (SSPE)
- Delayed sequelae to measles infection
- Progressive deterioration of mental and motor function
- High level of measles in serum.

Progressive Multifocal Leukoencephalopathy
- Demyelinating disease
- In elderly person whose immune response is impaired
- Deterioration of motor function, vision and speech
- Electron microscopy from culture shows polyomavirus-JC virus

Very Difficult to Kill Prions Inactivated by
- Autoclaving 134 °C for 4–5 hrs.
- Sodium hypoclorite, phenol, ether.

Diagnosis
- Clinical features, EEG, MRI
- Confirmed usually – Postmortem
- Western blot for prion detection in CJD.

36 Miscellaneous Viruses

ROTAVIRUS

- Belongs to family reoviridae
- Non-enveloped dsRNA viruses in II segments

Morphology

- Resembles wheels with short spokes – electron microscopy
    Usually double shelled capsid
    7 gps A-G. gp A-Most common

Epidemiology

- Commonest cause of diarrhea in infants and children
    Below age 5 years (6–24 month frequent)
    Mode – feco-oral route
    In adults – Adult diarrhea rotavirus (ADRV)

Clinical Features

- Vomiting IP 2-3 days
    Diarrhea
    Little or no fever
    Stools: Greenish yellow on pale with no blood or mucus
    Self-limiting: Recovery 5 to 10 days.

Pathogenesis

- Destruction of mature enterocytes in villous epithelium of SI
- Enterotoxin.

Lab Diagnosis

- **Specimen:** Feces, blood
- **Electron microscopy and immunoelectron microscopy**
    - Concentration more than 10^6 viruses/ml necessary.
- **Serological techniques**
    - IgM and IgG antibodies in blood – only epidemiological purpose
    - Demonstration of viral antigen in stools – most common method.

- Molecular diagnosis: PCR
- **Treatment**: Supportive
- **Vaccine** Roteteq ⎫
           Rotarix ⎭ live attenuated vaccine given to children

Other Viruses Causing Diarrhea

- Norwalk Virus
- Adenovirus
- Astrovirus
- Coronavirus

RUBELLA (GERMAN MEASLES)

Caused by Rubella virus

Rubella Virus

- RNA Virus
- Pleomorphic spherical particle.

Pathogenicity

- Mainly infects children also all ages
- Mode of infection: Inhalation
- Incubation period: Two to three weeks

Clinical Features

- Generalized rash: 1st on face then spreads to other parts sparing palm and soles
- Non tender enlargement of posterior cervical glands.

Complications: Arthralgia and Arthritis Congenital Rubella.

Rubella in Pregnancy

- Rubella in very early pregnancy: Fetus die
- Rubella in 1st trimester: Congenital malformations
- Later:
  - Communication defects
  - Development retardation
- Classical rubella syndrome:
  - Cardiac defects
  - Deafness
  - Cataract
- Expanded rubella syndrome:
  - Hepatosplenomegaly
  - Thrombocytopenia purpura
  - Myocarditis
  - Bone lesions

Lab Diagnosis

Important in pregnant women

- Pregnancy — Virus isolation
  - Serology – ELISA
- Congenital rubella isolation – urine, throat swabs, CSF
- Serology

Prophylaxis
MMR Vaccine

- Rubella vaccine 27/3 live attenuated vaccine, given s/c
- Given to female of child bearing age.

CORONAVIRUSES

- Enveloped RNA viruses
- Club shaped or petal shaped peplomers
- 2 groups — Acid labile viruses
  - Acid stable viruses

Severe Acute Respiratory Syndrome (SARS)
- Caused pandemic in 2002–03
- Mode of infection: Inhalation of droplets or aerosols of patients
- Incubation period: Under 10 days.

Clinical Features
- Fever with cough or other respiratory symptoms
- Diarrhea
- Death due to respiratory failure.

Lab Diagnosis
- Early: RTPCR
- Later: Demonstration of rise in titer of antibodies (ELISA, IF)
- Culture: Verocells.

Prophylaxis
No specific prophylaxis or Treatment (highly mutable virus).

ONCOGENIC VIRUSES

Virus that produce tumor in natural host or animals or which produce malignant transformation of cells on culture.

Oncogenic DNA Viruses

- Papovaviruses
  - HPV16 and HPV18: Cervical cancer
  - Polyomavirus
  - Simian virus 40.

- Poxvirus: Molluscum contagiosum
- Adenovirus
- Herpes virus Epstein: Barr virus
- Hepatitis B virus
  - Hepatocellular carcinoma

Oncogenic RNA Viruses

- Retrovirus: Enveloped, spherical viruses
- Single stranded RNA molecules.

Classification

- Oncovirinae
- Spumavirinae
- Lentivirinae.

Types Based on Host Range

- Avian leukosis complex
- Murine leukosis complex
- Mammary tumor virus of mice
- Leucosis: Sarcoma viruses of other animals
- Human t cell leukemia (lymphotropic) viruses
  - Infect CD4 cells
  - Causes adult T-cell leukemia
  - Tropical spastic paraparesis.

Oncogenesis

- Genes which encode proteins which trigger transformation of normal cells into cancer cells
- Two types cell
1. Cellular
2. Proto-oncogenes
- Ef: V-src, V-ras.

Mechanism of Viral Ontogenesis

- Oncogenic DNA viruses:
  - Viral DNA integrated in host cell genome
  - Host cell—Malignant transformation
- Oncogenic RNA viruses – Two mechanism
  - Introducing oncogene
  - Alteration of cellular oncogene.

37 Picornaviruses

- Nonenveloped RNA viruses
- **Classification**
  - Enterovirus
  - Rhinovirus
  - Hepatovirus
  - Parechovirus.

ENTEROVIRUS

- Further classified to:
  - Poliovirus types 1-3
  - Coxsackie virus A types 1-2
  - Coxsackie virus B types 1-6
  - Echovirus types 1-34
  - Enterovirus types 68-78.

POLIOVIRUS

- Mainly cause polio
- Nonenveloped, positive dense single stranded RNA.

Pathogenesis

- **Source of infection**: Fecus, air droplets from carriers.
- **Mode of transmission:** Ingestion, feco-oral route, inhalation, conjunctiva.
- Virus ⟶ Enters ⟶ Multiplies in epithelial and lymphatic tissue ⟶ Enters blood (1° viremia) Reticuloendothelial system ⟶ Blood (2° viremia) ⟶ Anterior horn cells ⟶ AFP.
- Direct transmission to CNS occurs following Tonsillectomy.
- In CNS:
- Multiplies in neurons ⟶ Degeneration of Nissl bodies ⟶ Phagocytosed by macrophages.
- Mainly affect anterior horn cells causing flaccid paralysis rarely posterior horn.

Clinical Features

- **Inapparent infection:** Individuals develop seroconversion.
  - Incubation period 10 days.
- **Minor illness:** Lasts for 1–5 days.
  - Consist of fever, headache, sore throat and malaise.
- **Major illness:**
  - 3–4 day following minor illness
  - Fever returns, neck rigidity and other features of meningitis.
  - Indicates CNS involvement.
- **Nonparalytic poliomyelitis:** Disease does not progress beyond stage of aseptic meningitis.
  - If paralytic: Focally distributive, flaccid
  - Spinal, bulbar or bulbospinal

Factors Influencing Incidence of Paralysis

- Pregnancy
- Injection such as triple vaccines
- Tonsillectomy
- Muscle exertion during preparalytic stage.

Lab Diagnosis

a. **Specimen:** Feces (collected as per AFP surveillance programme–transported through reverse cold chain) Blood, CSF, throat swab

b. **Virus isolation**
  - Blood: During the first week
  - Throat swabs: Early stage of disease
  - Fecus: Up to 6 weeks
  - Due to intermittent excretions, 2 samples collected on seperate days

c. **Decontamination** by suitable process.

d. **Culture:** Tissue Culture

e. **Serology:**
  - Neutralisation by antisera
  - Compliment fixation test
  - ELISA.

Molecular Diagnosis

- Reverse transcriptase PCR
- Sequencing: To differentiate wild virus, OPV strain and vaccine derived poliovirus.

Prophylaxis

a. Passive immunization: Not reliable.
b. Active immunization:
   Salk's killed vaccine
   Sabin's live attenuated vaccine: Dosage and schedule (refer appendix-III).

Pulse Polio Immunisation Programme (PPI)

- Introduced in India in 1995
- For eradication of Polio.
- Mass administration of OPV on a single day to all children aged 0–5 years.
- 2 doses at an interval of 4–5 weeks.
- Possibility of attenuated virus circulating in community by spread to contact leads to indirect immunization (herd immunity)
- Inhibit circulation of wild type virus.

Objectives

- Less than 5 years immunized
- AFP to be reported and stool collected within 14 days
- High level of surveillance
- Performance of good mop-up operation.
  - Usually during the period of November to February.
  - Given regardless of previous immunization status.
  - Does not replace UIP.
  - Last reported case in India 13 JANUARY 2011, West Bengal
  - 2012 february 25th India striked off from list of polio endemic countries.

COXSACKIE VIRUS

- Single stranded RNA virus, nonenveloped.
- Based on pathological change produced in suckling mice → Group A / Group B

Group A
- Generalized myositis and flaccid paralysis.

Group B
- Focal paralysis and spastic paralysis
- Spread by feco-oral route.

Clinical Features

Group A
- Herpangina
  - Vesicular pharyngitis
  - Febrile pharyngitis, headache, vomiting, and abdominal pain
  - Small vesicles on fauces and posterior pharyngeal wall.
  - Break down to form ulcer.
- Aseptic meningitis
- Hand foot and mouth disease: Papulovesicular lesions on skin and oral cavity
- Minor respiratory infections.

Group B
- Bornholm disease/Epidemic pluerodynia
- Myocarditis and pericarditis
- Juveline diabetes
- Orchitis
- Transplacental and neonatal transmission
- Postviral fatigue syndrome.

Lab Diagnosis
- Sample: From lesions and fecus
- Isolation: Suckling mice
  - Tissue culture and serodiagnosis not predictable.

38 AIDS

HUMAN IMMUNODEFICIENCY VIRUS (AIDS)

- Enveloped, spherical virus, two ssRNA copies as genetic material.
- Causative agents of AIDS Subgroup – lentivirus Family – Retroviridae.
- **Viral genes**
  - gag gene – core and shell is formed.
    p^{15}, p^{18} and p^{24}.
  - env gene – envelope glycoprotein gp 160.
    gp 120 and gp 41.
  - pol gene – reverse transcriptase and other enzymes.
- Other nonstructural and regulatory genes are also present (tat, nef, vif, rev).

Antigen Diversity

- Based on molecular and antigenic differences two types
- HIV 1 and HIV 2
- HIV 1 has A to J subtypes (C is prevalent in India).

Pathogenicity

- Mode of infection: Blood and body fluids (sexual, parenteral, perinatal) of infected persons.
  - Virus binds to CD4 receptor with the help of gp 120
    - Primarily CD4 lymphocytes
    - 5–10% lymphocytes
    - 10–20% macrophages and monocytes.
  - Interaction with G coreceptor – CXCR4 – T-cell trophic starins
- CCR5 – Macrophage trophic strains.
  - Fusion of viral envelope with host cell membrane by exposing gp 41 in viral cell surface
  - RNA of virus released into cytoplasm of host cell after uncoating
  - Viral genetic material turns to DNA by RT enzyme and get intergrated in host cell (called provirus)
    - Lytic infection is initiated releasing progeny virions that affect other cells
    - Infected T4 cells lose their proper function IL–2, IFN-γ level reduced
    - Along with CMI, humoral immunity too is affected.

- Enormous B-cells are formed due to polyclonal activation causing hyper gammaglobulinemia (useless immunoglobulin)
- Monocyte macrophage function also affected
- CD4, CD8 ratio is reversed.

Clinical Features

- Natural evolution of HIV infection occurs in following stages
- Window period – 2-12 weeks – Period between acquisition of infection and period of antibodies
- Incubation period may vary.

Group I

- Acute HIV infection (3-4 weeks)
- 50% of people experience low grade fever, malaise, headache, lymphadenopathy, rash.
- But become positive during course: Hence seroconversion illness (acute retreoviral syndrome).
- P24 antigenimia can be demonstrated at beginning of this phase
- Decrease CD4 cells.

Group II

- Asymptomatic/latent infection (last up for several years)
- Positive for HIV antibodies and are infectious
- Long-term survivors or long-term nonprogressors: Those who escape from cilinical AIDS for about 15 years after HIV infection
- Virus multiplication goes on throughout
- CMI and humoral immunity limits the viral load but not completely
- So decreased viremia, almost normal CD4 cell.

Group III

- Persistant generalized lymphadenpoathy (PGL)
- Enlarged lymph nodes at least 1 cm diameter in two or more noncontiguous extrainguinal sites that persist for at least 3 months.
- Absence of any current illness or medication.

Group IV

- 'AIDS' related complex (ARS)
- Considerable immunodeficiency with opportunistic infections
- Fatigue, unexplained fever, persistant diarrhea, weight loss more than 10% of body weight.

Opportunistic Infections

- Subgroups A to E are present as per CDC, USA
  - **Parasitic**
    - Toxoplasmosis
    - Cryptosporidiosis

- Isosporiasis
- Generalized strongyloidiasis
- **Mycotic**
  - Pneumocystis jiroveci
  - Candidiasis
  - Cryptococcosis
  - Aspergillosis
  - Histoplasmosis.
- **Bacterial**
  - Mycobacterial infections
  - Salmonellosis
  - Campylobacter infections
  - Legionellosis.
- **Viral**
  - CMV
  - Herpes simplex.
- **Malignancies**
  - Kaposi sarcoma
  - Lymphomas.

AIDS

- End stage disease when CD4 count < 200/µl, p24 raised, antibodies reduced.
- Irreversible breakdown of immune defense mechanisms.
- Respiratory symptoms – Dry cough, dyspnea, fever
  - P.carinii and mycobacterium
- Gastrointestinal system – Oral thrush, herpetic stomatitis.
  - Hairy leukoplakia
  - Kaposi sarcoma
- CNS – Toxoplasmosis, cryptococcosis.
- Malignancies – HL and NHL.
- Cutaneous – herpes lesions, Candidiasis, Xeroderma, Seborrheic dermatitis.

Lab Diagnosis

- In India diagnosis according to NACO guidelines
- No test is carried out without prior content of patient
- Pre- and post-test counseling must be conducted to educate the patient.

Need for Diagnosis

- Diagnosing patients
- Monitoring of treatment
- Screening of blood and antenatal screening (mother and high-risk group).

1. Nonspecific Tests

- TLC: Leukopenia (lymphocyte < 2000/mm^3)
- T-cell subset assays (T4–T8).

- Thromocytopenia
- Increased IgG and IgA levels.
- Diminished CMI: Skin tests.

2. Specific Tests

Antigen detection:
- Virus antigen seen after 2 weeks of infection (i.e. window period).
- In infection like needle stick injury its appearance delays.
- Useful in persons recently exposed to risk of infection.

Virus isolation
- Isolated from peripheral lymphocytes.
- Cocultivation with patient's lymphocyte with uninfected lymphocytes in presence of IL2.
- Demonstration by presence of enzymes and antigens of virus.

PCR
- DNA PCR and RNA PCR.
- Complex and costly.

Detection during window period
- $p^{24}Ag$
- PCR
- Virus isolation (if able).

Antibody detection
- 2–8 weeks to months for antibodies to appear
- Once appeared they increase in titer in spectrum for next several months.
- IgM – 8–10 weeks and remaining IgG.

Screening Tests
- ELISA
- Rapid tests – cylinder or cassette ELISA
- Simple tests.

Supplementary Tests

1. Western blot test
- HIV proteins separated according to PAGE are blotted on nitrocellulose paper.
- These are reacted with test sera and with enzyme conjugated anti-human globulin
- Results: Position of band on strip indicates antigen with which antibody reacted. Negative WB – No bands corresponding to molecular weights of antigens.
  - Positive WB – HIV 1 – 2 of 3 bands (p^{24}, p^{41}, gp 160/120).
  - HIV 2 – gp 36 instead of gp 41.

2. Line Immune assays.

3. Immunofluorescence test.

Imp of p²⁴Ag

- Detection during window period
- Children (< 18 months) — ELISA of antibodies not useful.

Strategies for HIV Testing

Strategy I
- To screen blood/blood products organ, tissues, sperm
- Sample subjected to E/R/S and if positive discarded
- **Single test done – if positive discarded**
  If negative blood taken for transfusion.

Strategy II
- For surveillance and diagnosis if AIDS indication present.
- If positive in first ELISA second ELISA is done again and again positive then reported
- **2 tests done: Both has to be positive to term HIV +ve.**

Strategy III
- In asymptomatic individuals
- Third positive is reported
- **3 tests done: If all three positive-HIV +ve**
- **If any one –ve then indeterminate.**

Modes of Transmission

1. Sexual intercourse
2. Blood and blood products
3. Mother to baby
4. Tissue and organ donation
5. Injections and injury.

Treatment

- Treatment and prophylaxis of infections and tumors
- General management of immunosuppressive measures
- Specific anti-HIV agents
- HAART – highly active anti-retroviral therapy
- HAART started when CD4 count is < 350/µl.

PEP (Postexposure Prophylaxis)

- Started within 2 hours. Can be delayed up to 72 hours
- Basic regimen – NRTI (2)
  Zidovudine + Lamivudine daily 28 days
- Expanded regimen – 2NRTI + Protease inhibitor for 28 days
  Zidovudine + Lamivudine + Indinavir.

39. Introduction to Parasitology

Parasites: Living organisms, which depend on a living host for their nourishment and survival. They multiply or undergo development in the host. Parasite can be classified as:

- **Ectoparasite:** Inhabit only the body surface of the host without penetrating the tissue, e.g. lice, ticks, and mites
- **Endoparasite:** Lives within the body of the host, e.g. most of the protozoan and helminthic parasites
- **Free living parasite:** Live independent of the host.

Endoparasites further classified as:

- **Obligate parasite:** Cannot exist without a host, e.g. toxoplasma gondi and plasmodium
- **Facultative parasite:** Either live as parasitic form or as free living form.

40 Ameba

- Classified under unicellular protozoans
- Pseudopodia for locomotion and phagocytosis.

Classification
a. **Intestinal Ameba**, e.g. *entameba histolytica, Entameba hartmani*.
b. **Free living Ameba**, e.g. *naegleria fowleri, Acanthamoeba*, etc.

Entamoeba Histolytica
- Causes amebic dysentery and amebic liver abscess.

Morphology
- Three morphological forms
    a. Trophozoite
    b. Precyst
    c. Cyst

Trophozoite
- Vegetative or growing stage
- Irregular shape and uses pseudopodia for locomotion.

Precyst
- Round or oval form of parasite formed by extruding food vacuoles
- Formed before encystment and has chromatid bars and glycogen vacuoles.

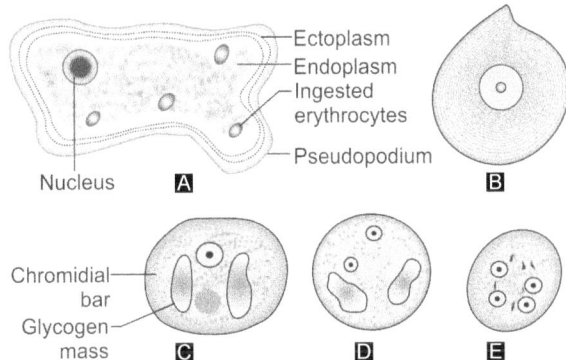

Figs 40.1 (A to E): Entamoeba Histolytica: A. Trophozoite **B.** Precystic stage **C.** Uninucleate cyst **D.** Binucleate cyst **E.** Mature quadrinucleate cyst

Cyst
- Spherical in shape
- Mature cyst – **Quadrinucleate.**

Life Cycle
- Life cycle in single host (called as **direct life cycle**)
- Infective form – Mature Quadrinucleate Cyst
- Mode of infection – Food and water contaminated with cysts.

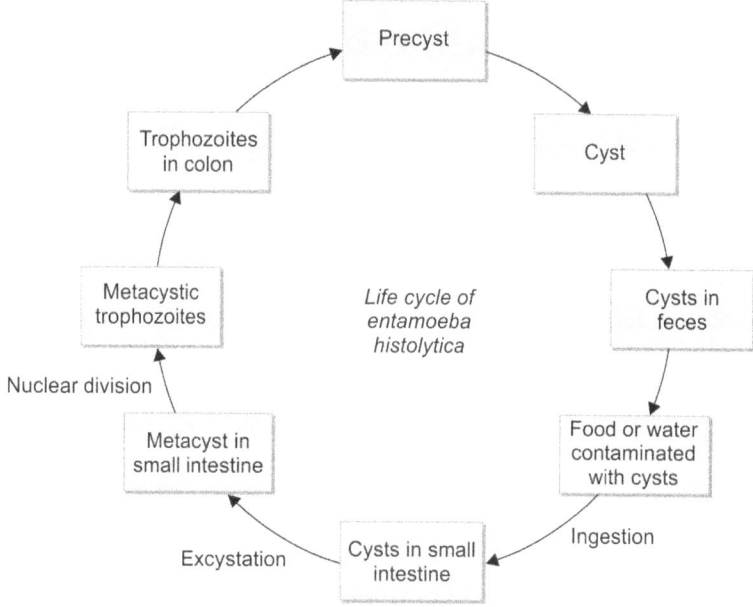

Fig. 40.2: Life cycle of entamoeba histolytica

Intestinal Amebiasis

Pathogenesis

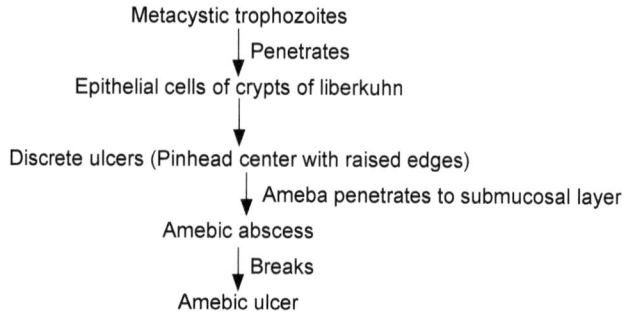

- Amebic ulcer – multiple, flask shaped in cross-section
- Breaks down to discharge brownish necrotic material.

Localized
- Ileocecal junction – Most common
- Sigmoidorectal region

Generalized

- Whole length of large intestine up to anal sphincter.

Clinical Features

- Typical manifestation—Acute amebic dysentery
- Passage of foul smelling brownish black stool with blood streaked mucus
- Sometimes diarrhea or abdominal symptoms like uncomfortable belly and growling abdomen are seen
- D/D – Bacillary dysentery.

Features	Amebic dysentery	Bacillary dysentery
Onset	Slow	Acute
Fever and tenesmus	Absent	Present
Stool		
Frequency	6-8/day	>10/day
Odor	Offensive	Nil
Nature and consistency	Mixed with blood and mucus, not adherent	Blood and mucus with little or no feces, adherent
Microscopy		
Eosinophil	Present	Absent
Charcot Leyden crystals	Present	Absent
Motile bacteria	Present	Absent
Ameba	**Motile trophozoites with ingested RBCs**	Absent

Extraintestinal Amebiasis

Hepatic amebiasis

- Most common extraintestinal complication
- Amebic hepatitis: Acute hepatic involvement due to invasion by ameba from colon
- Liver abscess (5–10%): Contain thick chocolate brown pus (Anchovy sauce pus).

Pulmonary amebiasis (very rare)

- Extension of liver abscess or hematogenous spread
- Chocolate brown sputum.

Metastatic amebiasis

- In kidney, brain, spleen, adrenals, etc.

Cutaneous amebiasis

- Genitourinary amebiasis

Lab Diagnosis

Intestinal Amebiasis
(a) Stool
Examination (i) Macroscopy – Blood and Mucus

(ii) Microscopy* (iii) Concentrated Method**

(b) Stool Culture
- NIH polygenic media
- Craig's medium
- Robinson's medium.

(c) Mucosal Scrapings

(d) Serology
ELISA

(e) Molecular
DNA probe

*Microscopy – In fresh stool of a/c amebic dysentery
- (a) Trophozoite with ingested RBC's
- (b) Motility

In Wet Film – Stained prepared cyst with
- (a) Iodine (glycogen mass stains brown)
- (b) Iron hematoxylin (Chromatin bodies – Jet black)

**Concentrated method
- Formol ether
- Zn Sulphate centrifugal floatation

Amebic Liver Abscess

- Microscopy
  - Trophozoite motility
  - Ingested RBCs
- Histopathology
  - Pus/aspirate
- Serology
  - ELISA
- Radiological
  - X-ray, CT, MRI
- Stool Examination for cysts

Treatment
- Luminal Amebicides – Diloxanidefuroate, iodoquinol
- Tissue Amebicides – Chloroquine, emetine
- Both – Metronidazole

Prophylaxis
- Health education
- Avoid stool contamination of food and water
- Detection and treatment of carriers.

PATHOGENIC FREE-LIVING 'AMEBA'

NAEGLERIA FOWLERI

- Causes Primary Amebic Meningitis (PAM)
- Habitat: Warm water

Morphology

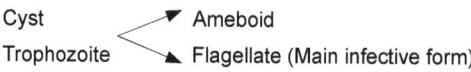

Cyst → Ameboid
Trophozoite → Flagellate (Main infective form)

Life Cycle
- Source of infection: *Swimming in fresh water*

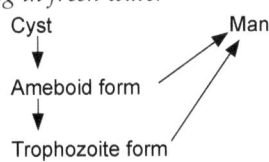

Pathogenesis and Clinical Features

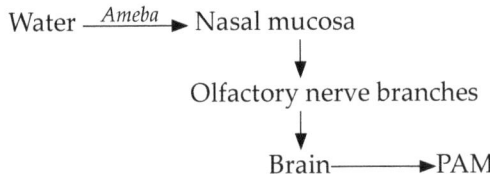

- Fever, headache, vomiting, neck stiffness, seizure
- Cranial nerve palsies.

Lab Diagnosis
- Resemble pyogenic meningitis

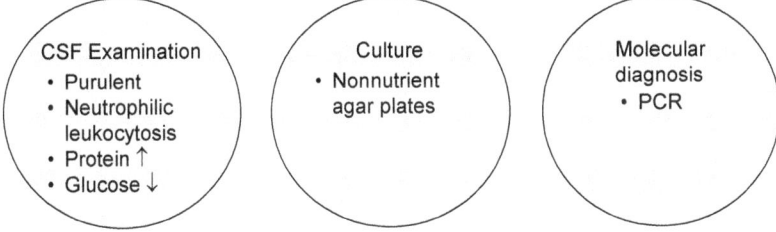

Treatment
- Drug of choice: IV amphotericin B.

ACANTHAMOEBA–(SPINE LIKE PSEUDOPODS)

- A. culbertsoni: Most common cause of human infection
- It causes – Chronic amebic keratitis (CAK)
  Granulomatous amebic encephalitis (GAE).

Distribution: Soil/water

Morphology
- Trophozoite form
- Cystic form.

Life Cycle
- Infective form: Cysts/Trophozoites
- Mode of infection: Inhalation/Ingestion of cysts.

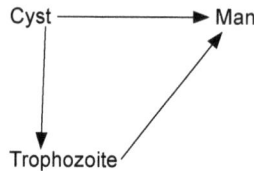

Pathogenesis and Clinical Features

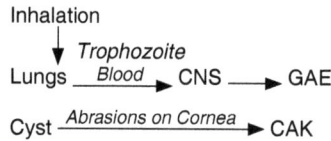

GAE: Seizures, paresis, mental deterioration.
CAK: Photophobia, redness, foreign body sensation.
- In contact lens users – Keratouveitis.

Lab Diagnosis

- Specimen
  - GAE – CSF
  - CAK – Corneal scrapings

- Amebic keratitis – Demonstration of cysts in corneal scrapings
- GAE – Demonstration of cysts/trophozoite in brain biopsy.

Treatment

- CAK – Biguanide and chlorhexidine ⟶ enucleation and corneal transplant
- GAE – No effective treatment.

41. Intestinal, Oral, and Genital Flagellates

Flagellates possess whip like flagella as their organs of locomotion.
2 types:

Lumen dwelling	Hemoflagellates
Found in alimentary tract and urogenital tract	
Example: Giardia lamblia	Example: Leishmania
Trichomonas	Trypanosomabrucci
Dientamebafragilis	Trypanosomacruzi
Enteromonashominis	

Giardia Lamblia

Two forms: 1. Trophozoite and 2. Cyst

Morphology

Trophozoites 14 × 7 μm	Cyst 12 × 7 μm
• Tennis racket or pyriform shape	Round /oval
• Dorsally convex, ventrally – concave sucking disc	2 pairs of nuclei axostyle forms a dividing line
• Bilaterally symmetrical	
- 1 pair of nuclei - 4 pairs of flagella - 4 pairs of blepharoblast - 1 pair of axostyle and 2 parabasal bodies	

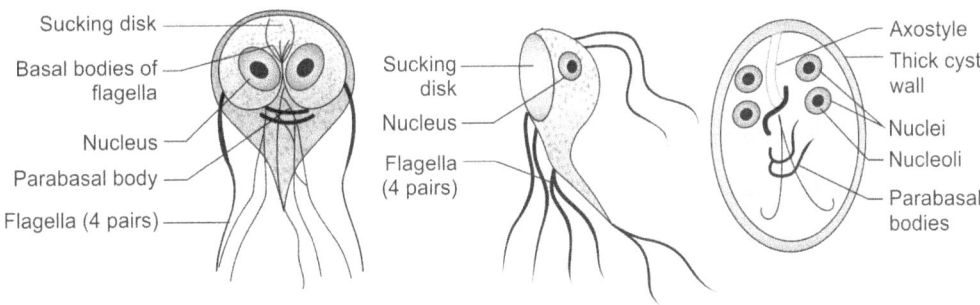

Fig. 41.1

Life Cycle

- **Habitat**: Duodenum and upper jejunum
- **Host**: Direct life cycle
- **Infective form**: Cyst
- **Mode of Infection**: Ingestion of cysts.

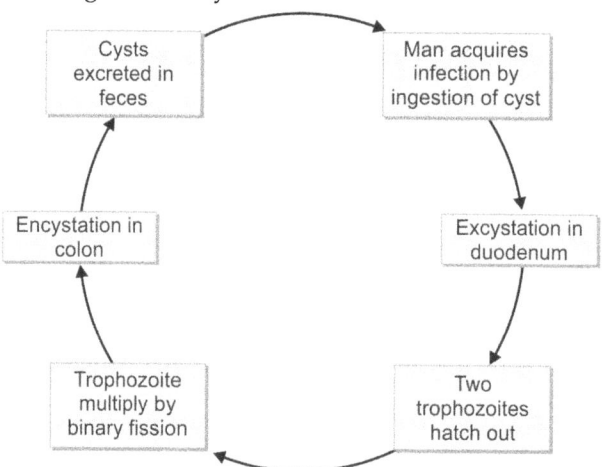

Pathogenicity and Clinical Features

Does not invade intestinal tissues
Adheres to intestinal epithelium

Causes abnormalities in villous architecture by cell apoptosis

Mucus diarrhea, malabsorption of fatty acids (leads to steatorrhea)
Epigastric pain and flatulence
May colonise gall bladder and cause biliary colic and jaundice

Lab Diagnosis

Stool examination	Enterotest	Serodiagnosis
1. Macroscopy Offensive odor, pale color, fatty, floats in water **2. Microscopy** Cyst and trophozoite	Gelatin capsule with coiled Thread ↓ Free end attached to cheek and swallow ↓ Passes to duodenum through Stomach ↓ Withdraw after 2 hours ↓ Placed in saline and centrifuged	**1. Antigen detection** ELISA, Indirect IF, Immunochromatography **2. Antibody detection** ELISA

Treatment

- Metronidazole 250 mg thrice daily × 5 days
- Tinidazole 2 gm once daily

Code of 2

- 2 Forms
- 2 Nuclei in trophozoite
- 2 axostyles
- 2 parabasal bodies
- 2 nuclei in young cyst
- 2 weeks incubation period
- 2 trophozoites hatch from cyst
- 2 lakh cyst in 1gm feces
- 2 hrs for enterotest.

Trichomonas

Three Species:
1. T. vaginalis
2. T. hominis
3. T. tetanax

Morphology

- Trophozoite only; no cyst form
    - Pear shaped with undulating membrane
    - 4 anterior flagella; 5th forming the undulating membrane that is supported by costa
    - Axostyle projects posteriorly as tail.

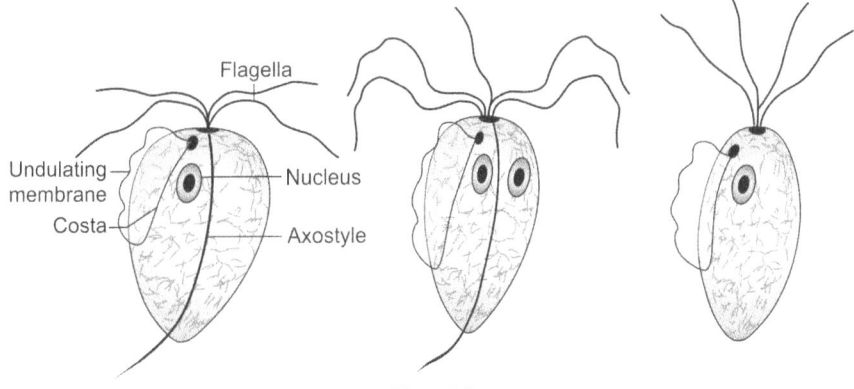

Fig. 41.2

Life Cycle

Habitat: Vagina, urethra, prostatic tissue
Infective form: Trophozoite
Mode of transmission: Person to person,
- Sexually transmitted usually
- Through fomites.

Pathogenesis

- Mainly infects squamous epithelium
- Causes petechial hemorrhage, metaplastic changes and desquamation of vaginal epithelium
- Leading to intracellular edema (chicken like epithelium).

Clinical Features

Males	Females	Infants
• Urethritis	• Pruritic vaginitis	• Conjunctivitis
• Epididymitis	• Yellowish green frothy discharge	• Neonatal pneumonia
• Prostatitis	• Dysuria	

Lab Diagnosis

Microscopy	Culture	Serology	Molecular
Wet Film of discharge shows jerky motility	Gold standard. More sensitive	ELISA	PCR
Stained with acridine orange Papanicolaou and giemsa stain			
Direct fluorescent antibody			

Treatment

Metronidazole: 2 gm single dose/500 mg orally twice a day for 7 days for both the partners.

42. Cryptosporidium Parvum

Diarrhea causing sporozoa: HIV related diarrhea

Morphology

- Oocyst: Spherical/oval
    - Two types: Thin walled: Causes autoinfection
                 Thick walled
    - Contains 4 sporozoites

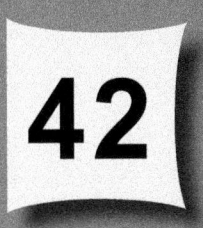

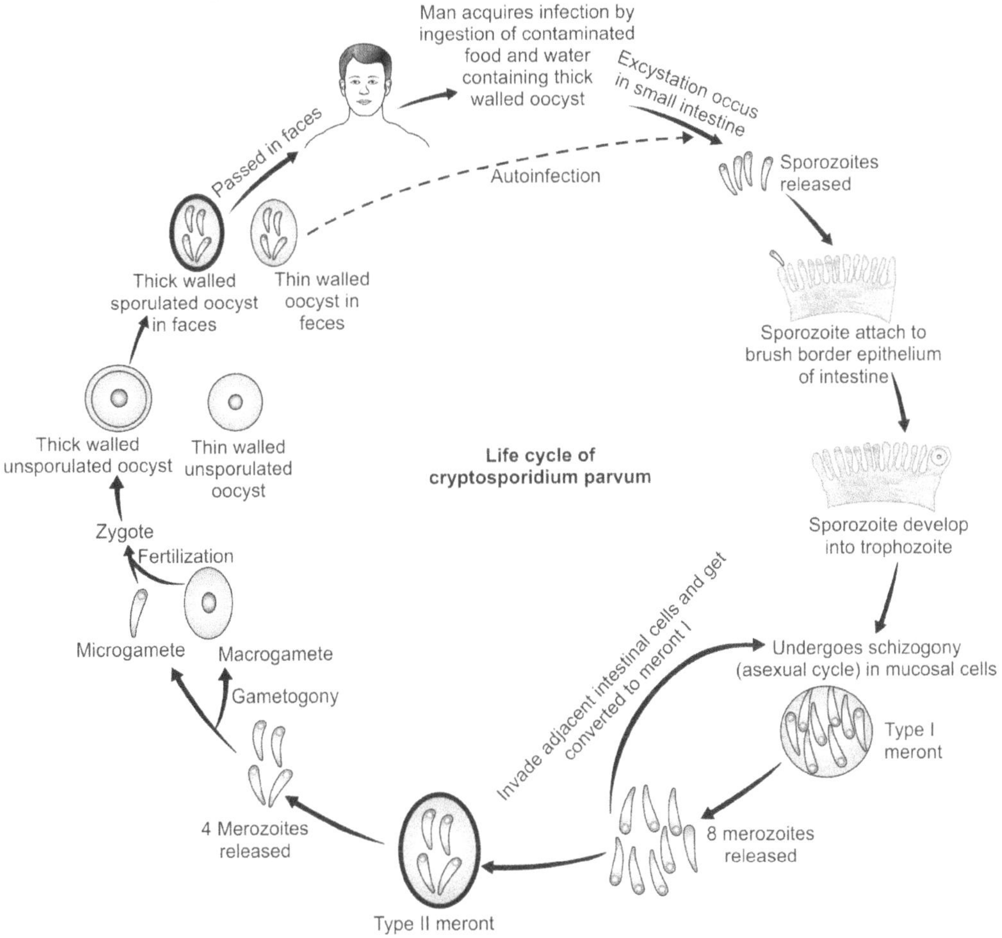

Fig. 42.1: Cycle of cryptosporidium parvum

Life Cycle

- **Habitat:** Small intestine, intracellular
- **Host:** Man
- **Infective form:** Oocyst
- **Mode of transmission:** → Ingestion of food and water with oocyst
  ↘ Autoinfection

Pathogenicity

- **In immunocompetent:** Asymptomatic/cause self-limiting febrile illness, watery diarrhea, abdominal pain, nausea and weight loss
- **In immunocompromised:** Chronic, persistent, profuse diarrhea Fluid and electrolyte depletion, weight loss, emaciation, abdominal pain.

Lab Diagnosis

1. Stool examination

Demonstration of oocyst

Staining:
- Cold Ziehl Neelsen stain: Internal structure appears acid fast
- Jenner–Giemsa stain: Oocyst appears as blue spherical bodies containing eosinophilic granules
- Fluorescent staining: With auramine phenol
- Indirect immunofluorescence: Using specific antibodies.

2. Histopathological examination

3. Serodiagnosis

ELISA: For antigen detection using monoclonal antibodies.

4. Molecular Diagnosis: PCR.

Treatment

No chemotherapeutic agent.

43 Pneumocystis Jirovecii

- It is saprophytic organism
- Also as an extracellular parasite in pulmonary alveoli
- Opportunistic infection-In immunocompromised patients.

Morphology

- **Trophozoite:** Ameboid with central nucleus
  — Divides by binary fission
- Cyst: Spherical with thick shell
- Has 8 oval shaped sporozoites.

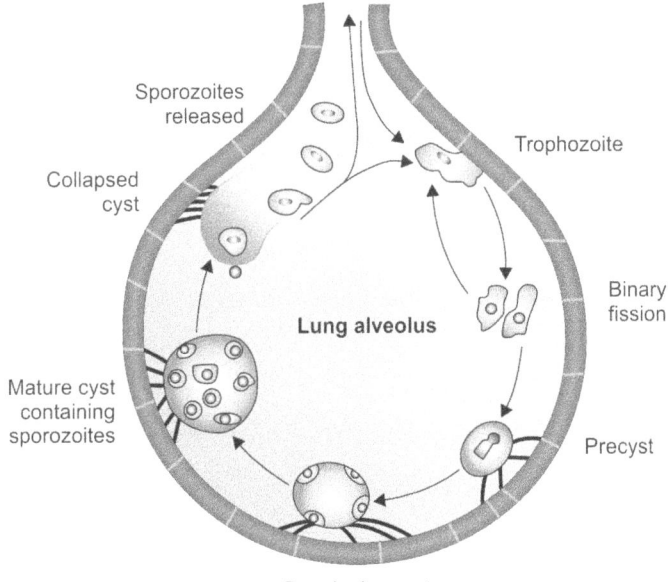

Fig. 43.1: Life cycle of pneumocystis jirovec G2

Life Cycle and Pathogenesis

- **Infective form:** Cyst
- **Mode of infection:** Spread by respiratory droplets
- It attaches to type-I pneumocytes resulting in alveolar damage

- A typical foamy vacuolar exudate is seen in alveoli on H and E staining
- Severe disease: Honey comb pattern with interstitial edema.

Clinical Features

- Nonproductive cough, dyspnea, high fever
- Involvement of liver, spleen and kidney (< 3%)
- Disease progression is rapid in immunocompromised patients
- Complication: Pneumothorax.

Lab Diagnosis

(GMS-Gomorimethanamine silver; PAS-Periodic acid Schiff)

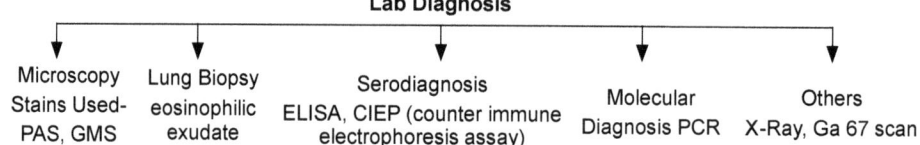

Treatment

- Trimetroprim–Sulfamethoxazole
- Pentamidine.

44 Coccidia

TOXOPLASMA GONDII

- Obligate intracellular coccidian
- Frequent association with HIV infection.

Morphology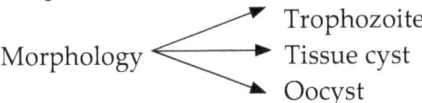
- Trophozoite
- Tissue cyst
- Oocyst

Trophozoite

- Crescent shaped
- Invade any nucleated cell
- Replicate in vacuoles (Endogony)
- Rapidly replicating trophozoites (tachyzoites).

Tissue Cyst

- Resting form of parasite
- Slowly replicating (bradyzoites).

Oocyst

- Develop only in definitive hosts
- Give rise to 2 sporocysts which obtains 4 sporozoites.

Life Cycle

- Definite host: cats (Enteric cycle)
- Intermediate host: Man and other mammals (Exoenteric cycle)
- Mode of infection: Ingestion of infective oocyst.

Pathogenicity and Clinical Features

- Congenital toxoplasmosis
  - From mother to fetus
  - Most are asymptomatic at birth
  - Manifestations – chorioretinitis, cerebral calcification, convulsions, microcephaly, hydrocephaly
- Acquired toxoplasmosis
  - Through ingestion reaches intestine
  - Cervical lymphnodes affected

- Mild flu
- Typhus like exanthema
- Ocular Toxoplasmosis – Uveitis, choroiditis, or chorioretinitis.

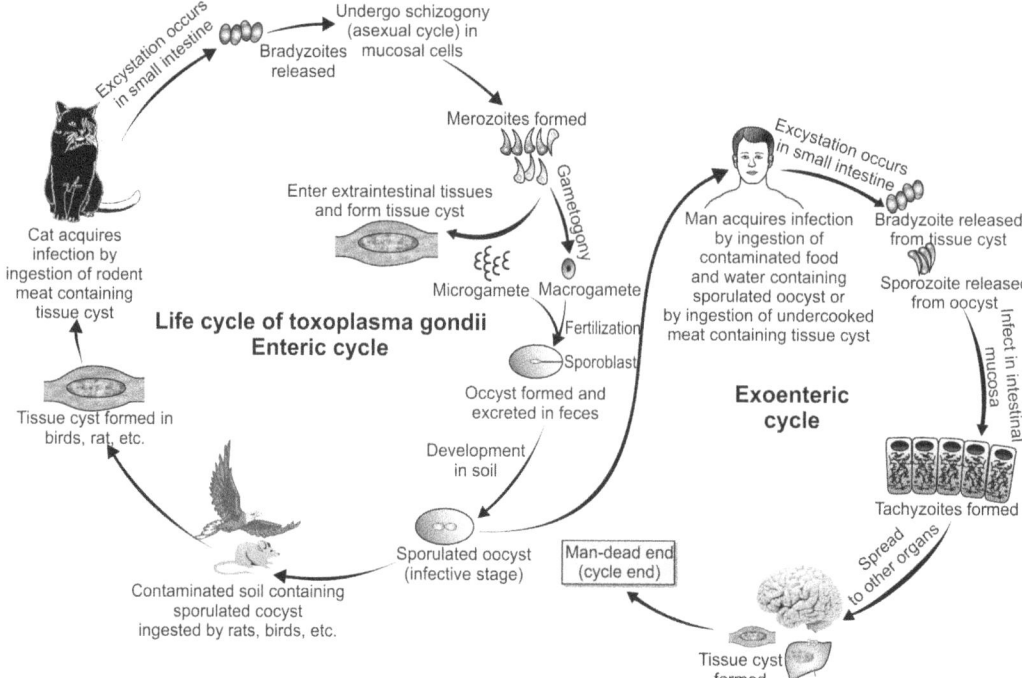

Fig. 44.1: Life cycle of toxoplasma gondii

Lab Diagnosis

- Microscopy of blood and sputum: Tachyzoites and tissue cysts are detected
- Serology: Sabin Feldman dye test
  - IgM ELISA
  - IgA ELISA
- Molecular diagnosis: PCR
- Imaging: CT and MRI for CNS involvement
- Others: Animal inoculation and Frenkel's test.

Treatment

- Congenital: Oral pyrimethamine + Sulfadiazine + Folinic acid for 1 Year
- Ocular: Oral pyrimethamine + Sulfadiazine for 1 month
- Immunocompetent: Trimethoprim – sulfamethoxazole is the DOC.

PROPHYLAXIS

- Individuals at risk (pregnant women, immunecompromised) should avoid contact with cat and its feces
- Proper cooking of meal and proper washing of hands, fruits and vegetables.

45 Malaria

- Malaria is a protozoal disease caused by Plasmodium spp.

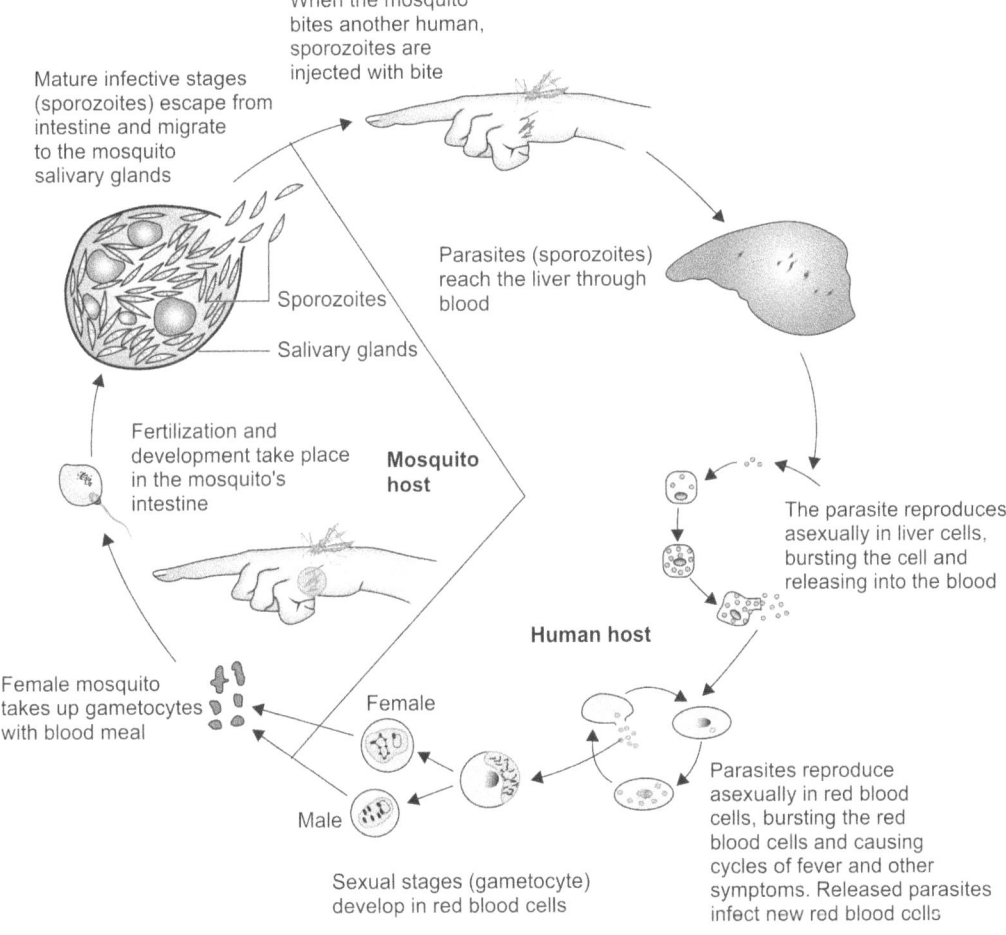

Fig. 45.1

Causative Agents

- Plasmodium vivax: Benign tertian malaria
- Plasmodium falciparum: Malignant tertian malaria

- Plasmodium malariae: Benign quartan malaria
- Plasmodium ovale: Ovale tertian malaria.

Vector

- Female Anopheles mosquito.

Life Cycle

- Definitive host: Female Anopheles mosquito
- Intermediate host: Man (mode of infection—mosquito bite)
- Human cycl: Schizogony and Gametogony – Asexual cycle
- Mosquito cycle: Sporogony – Sexual cycle
- Schizogony: Multiplication of malarial parasite by division < Erythrocytic / Exoerythrocytic
- Merozoites: Products of schizogony
- Hypnozoites: Sporozoites which become dormant in hepatocytes (P. vivax and P. ovale).

Pathogenesis

- All clinical manifestations are due to products of erythrocytic schizogony and hosts reaction to them
- Liver: Hepatomegaly, fatty changes, centrilobular necrosis
- Spleen: Splenomegaly, slate grey/brown/black color
- Kidneys: Enlarged and congested (Hemoglobinuric nephrosis)
- Brain: Encephalopathy
- Heart: Congestive cardiac failure
- Anemia.

Clinical Features

- Three important features are
  - Periodic fever—Because erythrocytic schizogony is synchronous ⟶ Release of waste products ⟶ Macrophages engulf released waste products and merozoites Release IL-1 and TNF ⟶ Acts on thermoregulatory center in brain
  - Anemia—Normocytic normochromic
  - Splenomegaly.
- Febrile paroxysm – 3 stages < Cold stage (chill) / Hot stage (Fever) / Sweating stage
- Periodicity
  - 48 hours – P. vivax P. falciparum
  - 72 hours – P. malaria

Malignant Tertian Malaria (P. falciparum)

- Cerebral malaria
  - Common cause of death
  - Due to capillary plugging.

- Blackwater fever – Malaria hemoglobinuria *(massive intravascular hemolysis by antierythrocytic auto antibodies)*
- Algid Malaria – Peripheral circulatory failure
  – Cold clammy skin
- Septicemic Malaria **Merozoite Induced Malaria**
- Transfusion malaria – Accidentally by transfusion of blood infected with malaria Relapse doesnot occur and IP is short
- Congenital malaria – Vertical transmission
- Renal transplantation
- Shared syringes.

Tropical Splenomegaly Syndrome

- Abnormal immunological response to malaria in endemic areas
  — IgM auto antibody kills CD8 cells
  — No suppressor activity ↓
  — SoB cells produce lots of IgM with no useful function
- Enormous splenomegaly and high titres of circulation of antimalarial antibodies with no parasites in peripheral smear
- Hypergammaglobulinemia and anemia are seen
- Changes occurs in liver, bone marrow, kidneys and adrenals
- Responds to antimalarial treatment.

Lab Diagnosis

- *Blood Smear–* Gold Standard
  (refer pathology)   *Thin smear – Determine the species
              *Thick smear – Sensitive

Quantitative Buffy Coat (QBC) Test

- New simplified method for diagnosing malaria
- Small quantity of blood is spun in QBC centrifuge
- RBC containing malarial parasite are less denser than normal RBC's and concentrate just below buffycoat of leucocytes
- Faster and more sensitive than thick blood smear
- Less sensitive and expensive than thin blood smear.

Microconcentration Technique

- Blood sample collected in microhematocrit tube is centrifuged at high speed
- **Serodiagnosis** – IFA and ELISA
- **Molecular** – DNA probe and PCR.

Newer Methods

  — Flourescence microscopy
  — Rapid antigen detection (Parasite F test)
  — Dual antigen test (Parasite LDH).

Other tests

  — Measurement of hemoglobin and packed cell volume
  — Total WBC and platelet count

- Measurement of blood glucose
- Coagulation test
- Urine for free hemoglobin
- Blood urea and serum creatinine

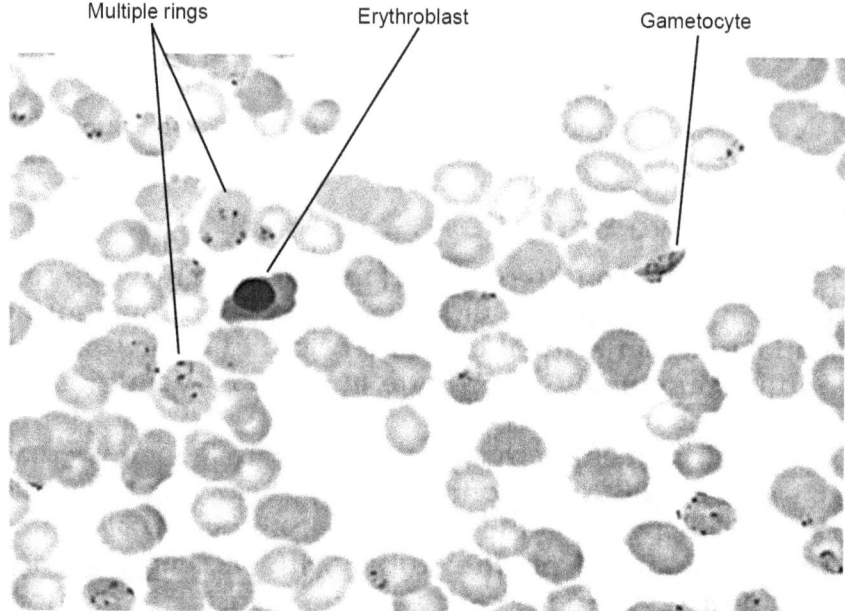

Fig. 45.2

Treatment

- Uncomplicated malaria
    Primaquine – 0.25 mg/kg – 14 days
        +
    Chloroquine – 25 mg/kg – 3 days
- Complicated malaria
    Chloroquine sensitive
    Chloroquine – 25 mg/kg – 3 days
        +
    Primaquine – 45 mg single dose
    Chloroquine Resistant (P.falciparum)
    ACT (Artemesinin Combined therapy)
    ACT + Sulphadoxime + Pyrimethamine

HEMOFLAGELLATES

TRYPANOSOMA BRUCEI GAMBIENSE (WEST AFRICAN TRYPANOSOMIASIS)

- Lives in man and other vertebrates
- Essentially a parasite of connective tissue also invades lymph nodes.

Morphology
- Vertebrate forms: Trypomastigote form
- Insect forms: In two forms
  1. Epimastigote
  2. Metacyclic trypomastigote forms

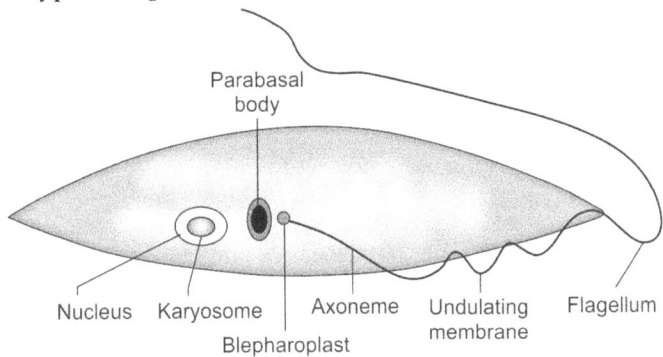

Fig. 45.3

Life Cycle
- Vertebrate host: Man, domestic animals
- Invertebrate host: Tsetse fly
- Infective form: Metacyclic trypomastigote form
- Mode of infection: Bite of tsetse fly, congenital transmission.

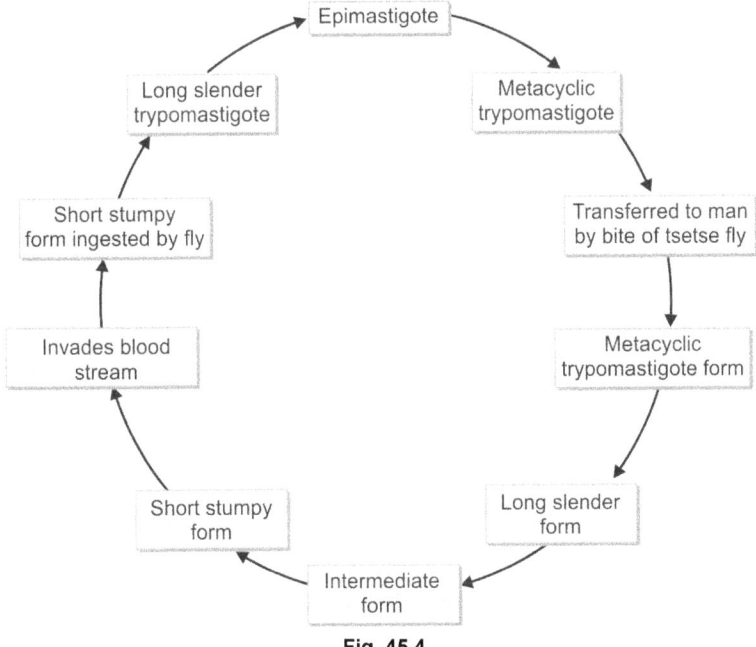

Fig. 45.4

Pathogenicity and Clinical Features
- Chronic illness
- Painless chancre at the site of bite

- Followed by fever, chills, rash, anemia
- Stage 1 disease: no CNS involvement
  - Hepatosplenomegaly, lymphadenopathy
  - Myocarditis, hematological manifestations. } HA staging
- Stage 2 disease : CNS involvement
  Sleeping sickness.

Lab Diagnosis

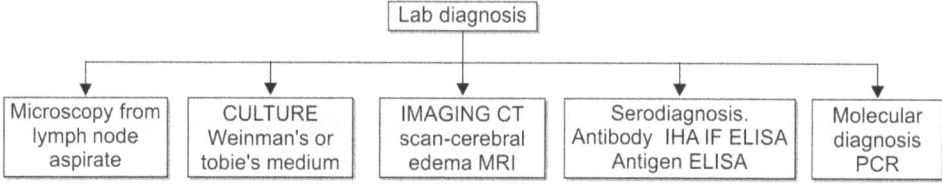

TRYPANOSOMA BRUCEI RHODESIENSE

- More acute than West African sleeping sickness
- Myocarditis and febrile paroxysms more prominent
- Lymphadenitis less prominent.

TRYPANOSOMA CRUZI

- Causative organism of Chaga's disease
- In humans – exist in amastigote and trypomastigote forms
- In reduviid bugs – amastigote and metacyclic trypomastigote.

Morphology

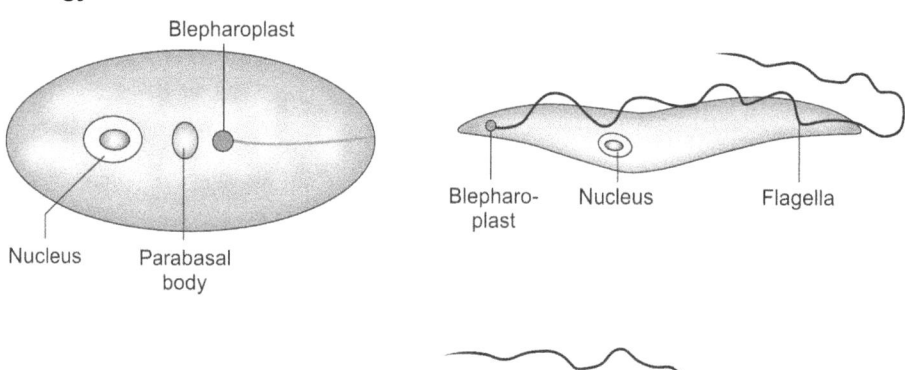

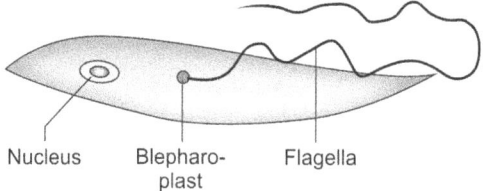

Fig. 45.5

- Amastigote: Oval bodies
    - Kinetoplast and nucleus present
- Trypomastigote: Long, thin, flagellates
    - Or short stumpy form
    - Do not multiply in humans
- Epimastigote: Kinetoplast adjacent to nucleus
    - Undulating membrane seen.

Life Cycle

- Definitive host: Man
- Intermediate host: Reduviid bug (vector)
- Reservoir host: Armadillo, cat, dog
- Infective form: Metacyclic trypomastigote.

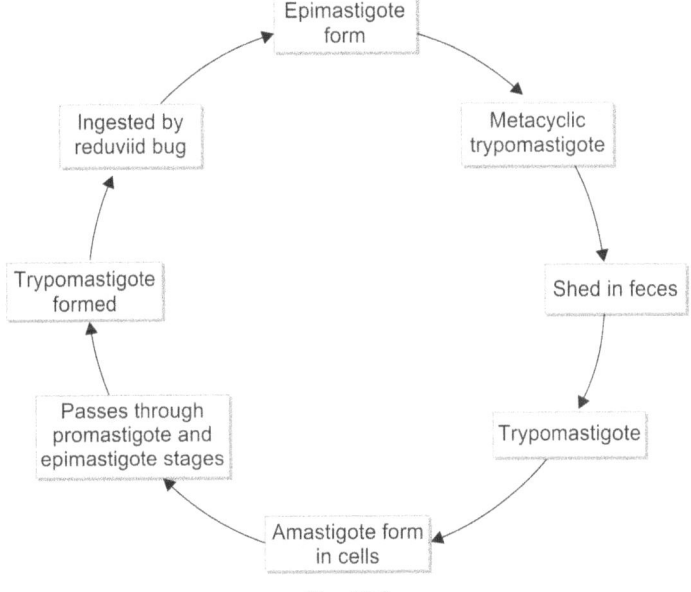

Fig. 45.6

Pathogenicity and Clinical Features

- Acute Chaga's disease:
    — Children < 2 years
    — 'Chagoma': Subcutaneous lesion at site
    — In few fever, lymphadenopathy, hepatosplenomegaly
    — May die due to myocarditis, encephalitis
    — 'Romana's sign: Inoculation of organism into eye causes edema of periocular tissues'.
- Chronic Chaga's disease:
    — In adults and older children
    — Cellular destruction, muscle and nerve fibrosis
    — Loss of tone – heart, esophagus, colon (myopathy, megaesophagus, megacolon).

Lab Diagnosis

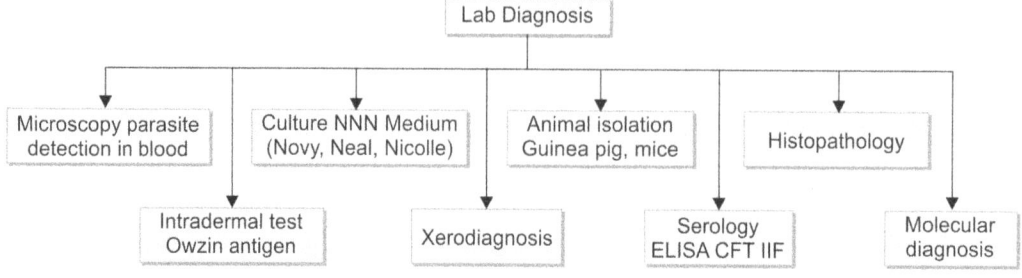

LEISHMANIA

- Obligate intracellular parasites
- Life cycle in 2 hosts – mammal and insect vector
- In human, resides within macrophage as amastigote form, as promastigote in invertebrate host.

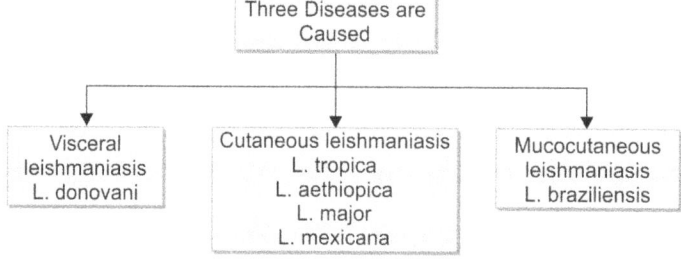

Leishmania Donovani

- Old world leishmaniasis
- Causes Kala-azar (Visceral leishmaniasis), Post Kala-azar dermal leishmaniasis (PKDL)
- Parasite of reticuloendothelial system (RES).

Morphology

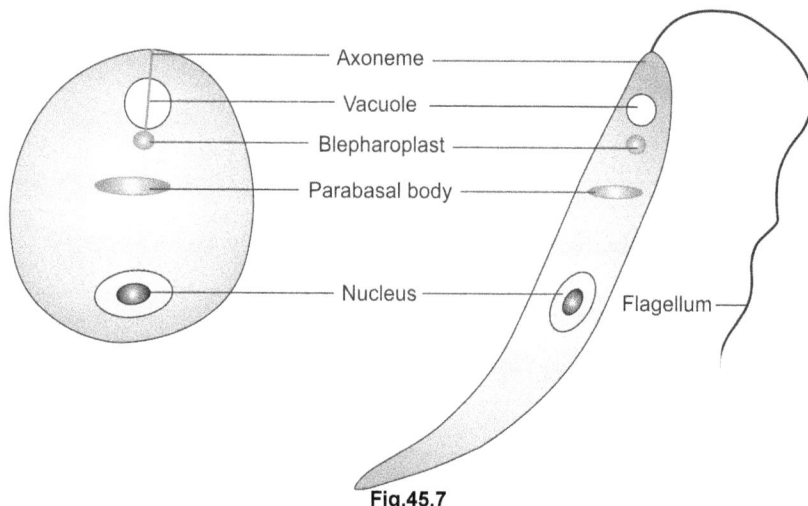

Fig.45.7

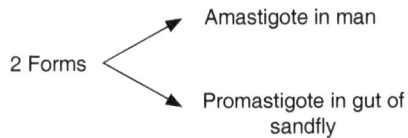

Amastigote	Promastigote
Ovoid/round cell, nonmotile	Long spindle shaped cells
Also known as LD bodies	No undulating membrane
Seen inside cell of RES	Seen in insect vector
Oval nucleus stains red	Central nucleus
Blue cytoplasm	Pale blue cytoplasm with red kinetoplast
Purple stained kinetoplast consisting of parabasal body and blepharoblast	Kinetoplast lies transversely
Flagellum absent	Single flagellum

Life Cycle

- Habitat: RES
- Definitve host: Man and other mammals
- Vector: Female sandfly
- Infective form: Promastigote within midgut of female sandfly
- Mode of transmission: Insect bite
- Vertically from mother to fetus.

Pathogenesis

- Multiplies in fixed macrophages and produce blockade of RES.
- Spleen—enlarged, capsule thickened
- Becomes soft and friable
  — C/S: 6 red or chocolate

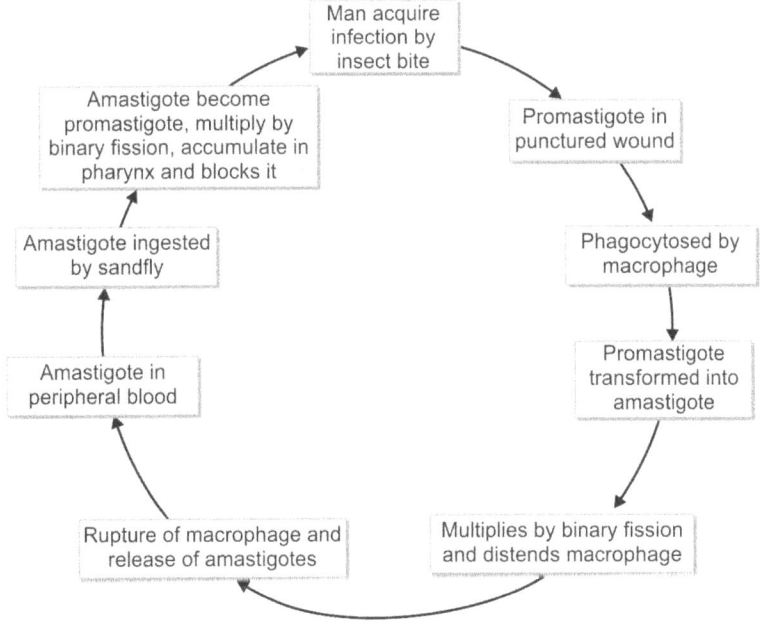

Fig. 45.8

- Liver: Liver function not affected but enlarged
  - C/S: nutmeg appearance
- Lymphadenopathy
- Severe anemia
- Bone marrow infiltrated with parasite.

Clinical Features

- Fever, hepatomegaly, splenomegaly
- Skin Dry, rough, darkly pigmented
- Cachexia and epistaxis.
- PKDL (Post kala-azar dermal leishmaniasis).

[3–10%]

- 1 or 2 year after recovering from systemic illness-3 types:
  a. Depigmented macules – on trunks and extremities
  b. Erythematous patches on nose, cheeks, and chin
  c. Yellowish pink nonulcerating nodules appear resembling that of leprosy.

Lab Diagnosis

Direct evidence

a. Microscopy: Gold standard

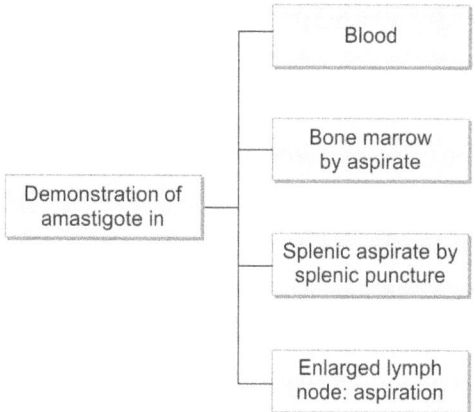

b. Blood: LD bodies within macrophage, monocytes, etc.
   - Buffy coat smear examined.
c. Culture: In NNN medium/Schneider's medium to demonstrate promastigote
d. Animal inoculation.

Indirect Evidence

a. Serodiagnosis
   - Detection of antigen – ELISA
   - Detection of antibody – CFT

DAT
 IFAT
 ELISA/DOT-ELISA
CIEP
b. Molecular Diagnosis: PCR
c. Nonspecific serum test
    — Aldehyde test
    — Chopra's antimony test.
d. Skin test
    — Monetenegro test
    — Delayed hypersensitivity test
    — 0.1 ml killed promastigote suspension injected ID on dorsoventral aspect of forearm
    — Induration and erythema of 5 mm or more after 48–72 hours
    — Positive – indicates prior exposure.
e. Blood picture
    — Pancytopenia
    — Reversal of A:G ratio.

Treatment

- Sodium stibogluconate–IV
- Amphotericin
- B Paromomycin
- Miltefosine.

46 Trematodes

- Unsegmented helminths, flat and broad parasites.
- Classification
  - Blood flukes
  - Liver flukes
  - Intestinal flukes
  - Lung flukes.
- **Morphology:**
  Two suckers: 1. Oral sucker surrounding the mouth
  2. Ventral sucker in the middle.
Reproductive system well developed- Monoecious/dioecious
Oviparous.

47 Intestinal Flukes

1. Fasciolopsis buski: Largest trematode infecting man
2. Heterophyes: Smallest trematode infecting man
3. Metaognimus yokogaweri
4. Watsonius watsoni
5. Echinostoma
6. Gastrodiscoides hominis

1–5 resides inside small intestine and 6 in large intestine.

FASCIOLOPSIS BUSKI

- Also known as Giant Intestinal Fluke
- Morphology:
  - Adult worm: Hermaphrodite worm
  - Egg: Operculated.

Similar to that of Fasciola hepatica.

Life Cycle

- Habitat: Duodenum/jejunum of pigs and man
- Definitive host: Pig and man
- First Intermediate host: Snail
- Second Intermediate host: Aquatic plants
- Infective form: Encysted metacercariae on aquatic plants.

Pathogenesis

- Initially diarrhea and abdominal pain
  - Traumatic: Inflammation and local ulceration due to attachment of larva to duodenal and jejunal mucosa
  - Mechanical: Partial obstruction of bowel
  - Malabsorption
    - Protein losing enteropathy
    - Impaired Vit B_{12} absorption
  - Toxic : Edema, ascites, anemia, and persistent diarrhea

Lab Diagnosis

- Stool microscopy: Eggs in feces
- Serodiagnosis.

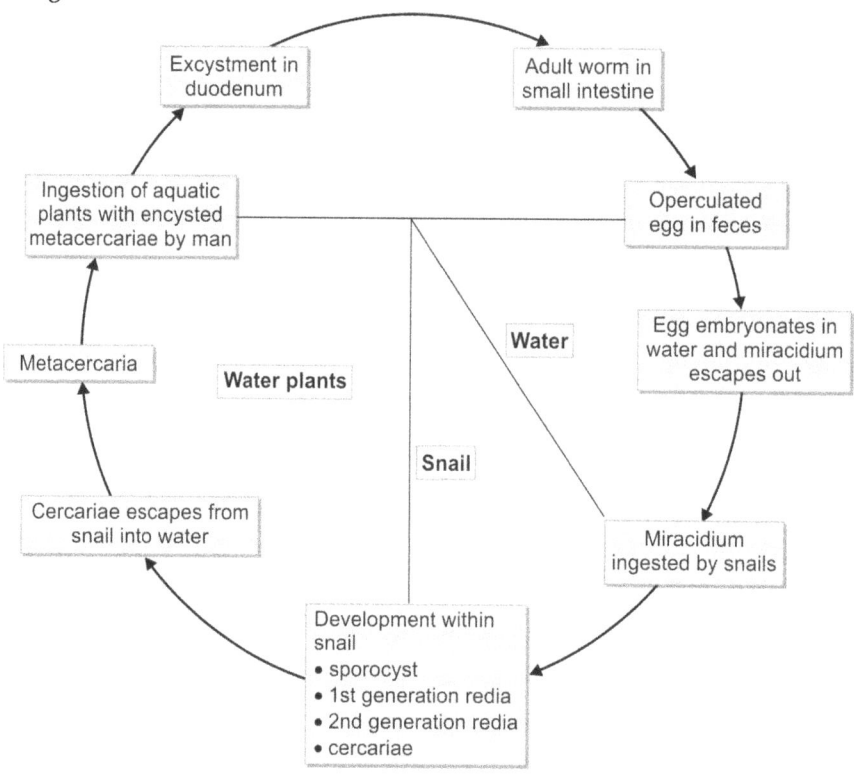

Treatment

- Praziquantel.

LUNG FLUKES

■ PARAGONIMUS WESTERMANI

- Egg:
  - Operculated
  - Bile stained.

Life cycle

- Habitat: Cystic spaces in lung
- Definitive host: Man and domestic animals
- First Intermediate host: Snail
- Second Intermediate host: Crab/Cray fish
- Infective form: Metacercariae encysted in crab/cray fish
- Mode of Infection: Eating under cooked crab/cray fish with metacercariae.

```
                    Penetrates intestine        Adult worm
                    and diaphragm               in lung

    Metacercariae excysts                       Operculated egg in
    in duodenum                                 sputum or feces
                          Man
                                        Water

    Man get infected by                         Egg embryonates in water and
    ingestion of crab                           miracidium released

                                  Snail
                                              Development within snail
    Metacercariae develops                      • sporocyst
    inside crab                                 • 1st generation redia
                                                • 2nd generation redia
                          Crab                  • cercariae

              Cercariae              Cercariae escapes
              penetrates crab        into water
```

Pathogenicity and Clinical Features

- **Pulmonary:**
  - Worm is cystic space lined by fibrous capsule
  - Perigranulomatous lesions, cystic dilations, abscess, hemoptysis
  - Eggs within sputum.
- **Extrapulmonary:**
  - Abdominal pain and diarrhea
  - Cerebran type: Resemble cysticercosis
  - Glandular involvement cause fever and multiple abscesses.

Lab Diagnosis

- Microscopy: Eggs in feces/sputum
- Serology: CFT, IF, ELISA, IHA
- Imaging:
  - X-ray: Abnormal shadow in middle and lower lung field
  - CT scan: Soap bubble like appearance in cerebral cysts.

BLOOD FLUKES/SCHISTOSOMES

- S. hematobium: Pelvic venous
- S. Mansoni: Inferior mesenteric vein
- S. Japonicum: Superior mesenteric vein.

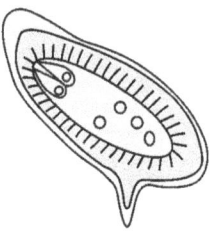
S. mansoni
Ova with a lateral spine
(obtained from stool)

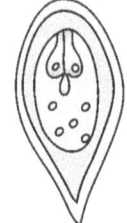
S. hematobium
Ova with a terminal spine
(obtained from urine)

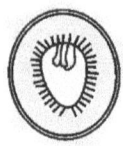
S. japonicum
Ova with a lateral knob
(obtained from stool)
Note: The characteristic surround
of tissue particles

Fig. 47.1: Schematic diagram to show distinguishing features of eggs of S. mansoni, S. hemotobium and S. joyponicum

- **Distinguishing features from others:**
  - Unisexual
  - Lack pharynx
  - Caeca unite after bifurcation
  - Nonoperculated egg
  - No redia stage
  - Cercariae have forked tails.

- **Egg:**
  - Nonoperculated, brownish yellow
  - Terminal spine
  - Egg laid one by one in vesical/pelvic plexus
  - Pass through vesical wall by action of spine
  - Discharged in urine.

Life Cycle

- Definitive host: Humans
- Intermediate host: Fresh water snails
- Infective form: Cercaria larvae
- Mode of infection: Cercaria penetrate to unbroken skin
- S. mansoni: Egg in feces
- S.japonicum: Egg in feces
- S.hematobium- egg in urine

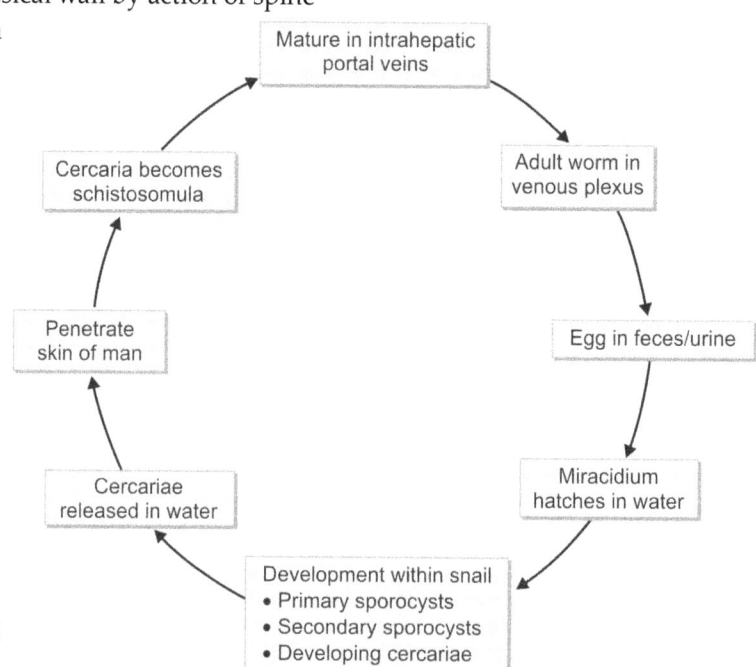

Pathogenicity and Clinical Features

- Depend on stages in evolution

Skin penetration and incubation period
    a. Cercarial dermatitis consisting of itching and petechial lesions (swimmer's itch)
    b. Anaphylactics symptoms like fever, headache, and malaise
    c. Leucocytosis, eosinophilia, hepatosplenomegaly.
- Egg deposition
  a. Hematuria
  b. Increased frequency of micturition
  c. Hyperplasia and inflammation of bladder.
- During tissue proliferation and repair
  a. Pseudo abscess at the site of deposition Chronic cystitis
  b. Bladder calculi
  c. Sandy Patch: Hyperplasia and fibrosis of vesical mucosa with granular appearance.

Lab Diagnosis

1. Demonstration of egg:
   a. Urine microscopy
   b. Bladder mucosal biopsy
2. Imaging:
   a. X-ray abdomen-bladder calculi seen
   b. USG
   c. Intravenous Pyelogram
   d. Cystoscope
3. Detection of antigen: by ELISA
4. Detection of antibody: CFT, IHA, ELISA, Immunofluorescence
5. Intradermal skin test (Fairley's test).

Treatment

- DOC- Praziquantel, Metriphonate.

LIVER FLUKES

- Clonorchis sinensis
- Fasciola hepatica

■ FASCIOLA HEPATICA (SHEEP LIVER FLUKE)

- Largest liver fluke
- Habitat–Liver and biliary passages.

Morphology

- **Egg:**
  - Large, ovoid operculated
  - Bile stained
  - Contain immature larva
  - Miracidium
  - Unembryonated when freshly passed.

Life cycle

- Definitive host: Sheep, goat, cattle, man
- Intermediate host: Snail
- 2nd intermediate host: Aquatic plants
- Most of infection: Ingestion of metacercariae encysted on aquatic plant.

As shown below, Fasciola parasite develop into adult flukes in the bile ducts of infected mammals, which pass immature fasciola eggs in their feces. The next part of the life cycle occurs in freshwater. After several weeks, the eggs hatch, producing a parasite from known as the miracidium, which then infects a snail host. Under optimal conditions, the development process in the snail may be completed in 5 to 7 weeks; cercariae are then shed in the water around the snail. The cercariae lose their tails when they encyst as metacercariae (infective larvae) on water plants. In contrast to cercariae, metacercariae have a hard outer cyst wall and can survive for prolonged periods in wet environments.

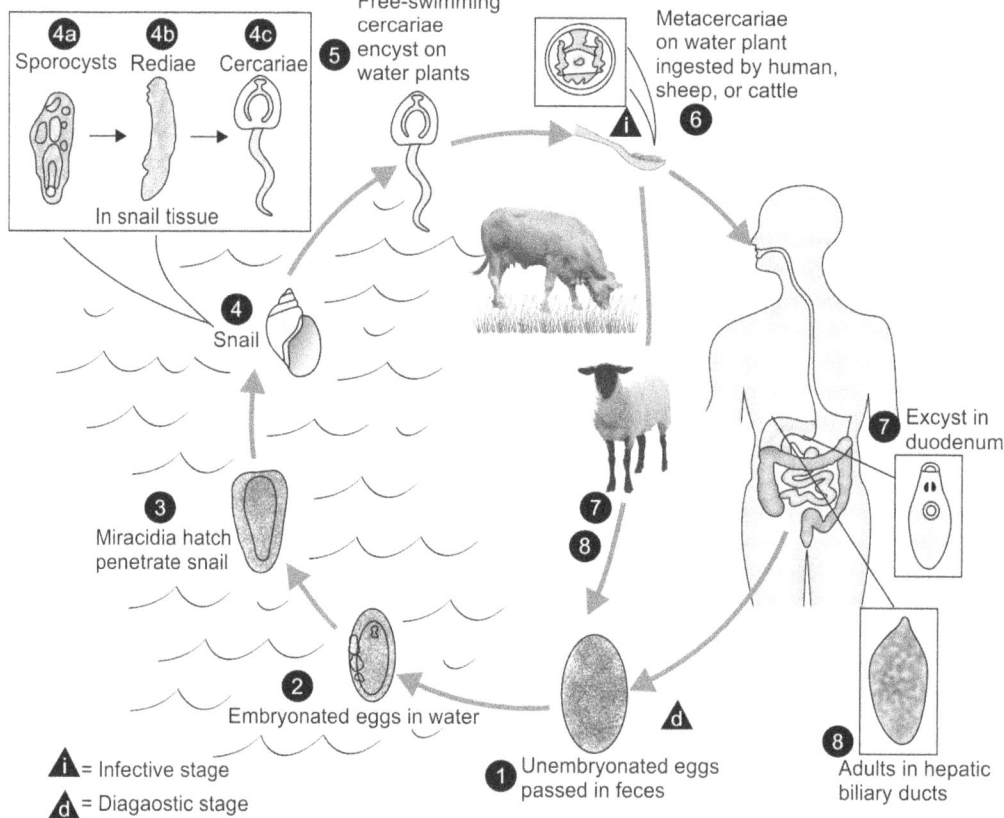

Fig. 47.2: 1. Immature Fasciola eggs are discharged in the biliary duct and in the stool, 2. Eggs become embryonated in water, 3. Eggs release miracidia, 4. Which invade a suitable snail intermediate host. Including the genera *Galba, Fossaria* and *Pseudosuccinea*, 4a. In the snail the parasites undergo several developmental stage (sporocysts), 4b. Rediae, 4c. Cercariae, 5. The cercariae are released from the snail, 6. Encyst as **metacercariae** on aquatic vegetation or Humans can become infected by ingesting, the metacercariae containing freshwater plants especially watercress, 7. After ingestion, the metacercariae excyst in the duodenum, 8. Migrate through the intestinal wall the peritoneal cavity, and the liver parenchyma into the biliary ducts, where they develop into adult flukes

In humans, maturation from *metacercariae* into *adult flukes* takes approximately 3 to 4 months. The adult flukes (*Fasciola hepatica*: up to 30 mm by 13 mm; *F. gigantica*: up to 75 mm) reside in the large biliary ducts of the mammalian host. *Fasciola hepatica* infect various animal species, mostly herbivores (plant-eating animals).

Pathogenesis and Clinical Features

Causes fascioliasis

- Acute phase:
  - Due to migration of larva
  - Fever, right upper quadrant pain
  - Eosinophilia and tender hepatomegaly
- Chronic phase:
  - Biliary obstruction
  - Biliary cirrhosis
  - Obstructive jaundice
  - Cholelithiasis, anemia
- Halzoun: Due to ingestion of raw liver of infected sheep.

$$\text{Adult worms attach to pharyngeal mucosa} \downarrow \text{Edematous congestion} \downarrow \text{Dyspnea, dysphagia, deafness}$$

Lab Diagnosis

- Stool microscopy: Egg demonstration
- Blood picture: Eosinophilia
- Serodiagnosis: IF, ELISA, CFT, Immunoelectrophoresis
- Imaging: USG, CT scan, Percutaneous cholangiography.

Treatment

- Oraltriclabendazole, Bithionol.

CLONORCHIS SINENSIS (ORIENTAL LIVER FLUKE)

Morphology

- **Egg:**
  - Oval and bile stained
  - Operculum at one end and knob at other end
  - Egg contains ciliated miracidia.

Life Cycle

- Habitat: Biliary passage/pancreatic duct
- Definitive host: Humans
- 1st Intermediate host: Snail
- 2nd Intermediate host: Fish

- Infective form: Metacercaria larva
- Mode of infection: Ingestion of undercooked fish carrying metacercariae.

Pathogenesis

- Due to larva:
  - Desquamation, hyperplasia and adenomatous changes of bile duct.
- Due to adult worm:
  - Cholangitis
  - Calculus formations
  - Biliary cirrhosis and portal hypertension
  - Cholangiocarcinoma:

Symptoms: Epigastric pain, fever, diarrhea, tender hepatomegaly.

Lab Diagnosis

- Stool microscopy
- Serological test: IF, ELISA, CFT
- Intradermal allergic test.

Treatment: Praziquantel

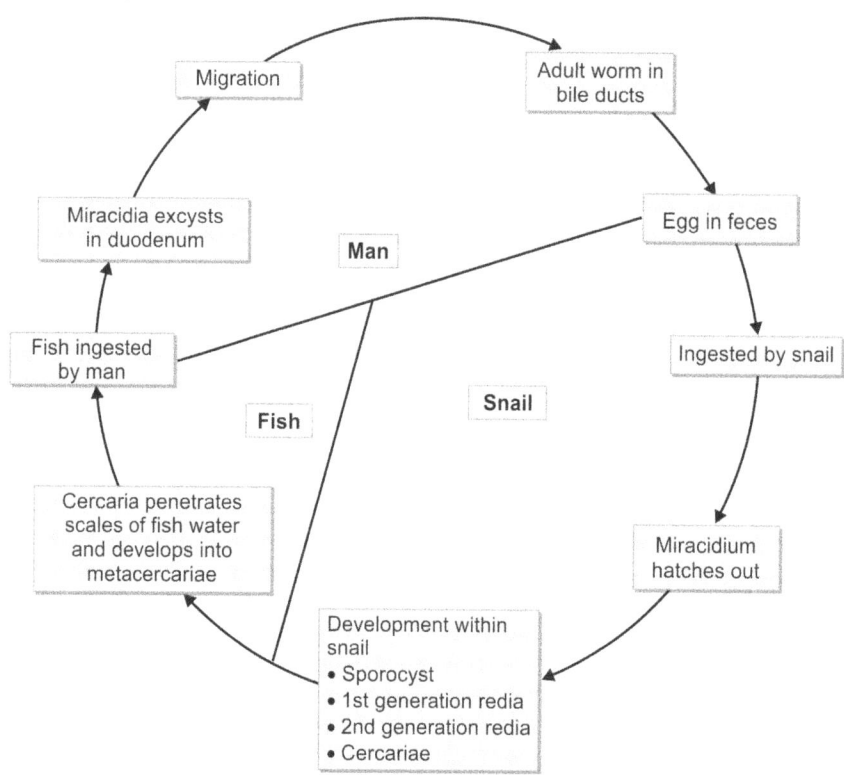

48. Cestodes (Tapeworms)

Two Classes

1. Pseudophyllidea: Diphyllobothrium latum
2. Cyclophyllidea: T. saginata
   T. solium

Hymenolepis nana

	Taenia solium	Taenia saginata	Hymenolepis nana	Hymenolepis diminuta	Diphyllobothrium latum	Echinococcus granulosus
Heads	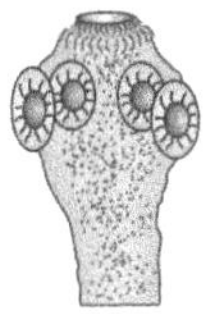	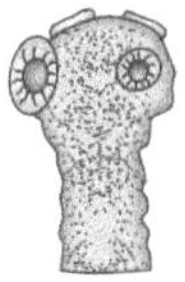	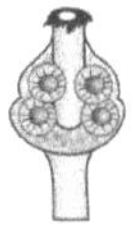	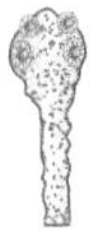	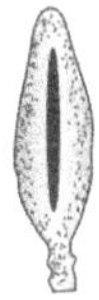	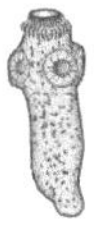
	4 Suckers 2 Rows of hooks	4 Suckers No hooks	4 Suckers single row of 20–30 hooks	4 Suckers No hooks	2 Suctorial grooves or bothria No suckers, No hooks	4 Suckers 2 Rows of hooks
Proglottids	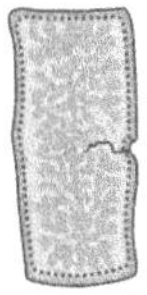	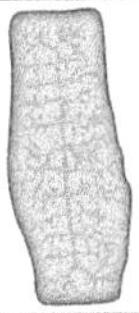	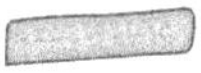	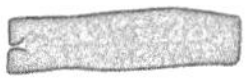	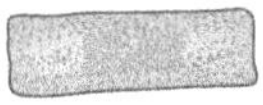	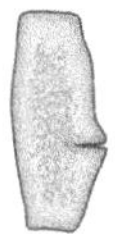
	Longer than broad 7–12 uterine branches on each side	Longer than broad 15–30 uterine branches on each side	Broader than long	Broader than long	Broader than long Uterus coiled	Longer than broad

Fig. 48.1

General Characteristics

- For every adult worm there will be three parts → Head (scolex)
  → Neck
  → Trunk (strobila)-proglottids

DIPHYLLOBOTHRIUM LATUM (FISH TAPEWORM)

- Longest cestode infecting human
- **Morphology:**
  - **Adult Worm:**
    - Scolex: It is spatulate/spoon shaped.
    - Bothria (2 slit like sucking grooves)
    - Neck: Thin, unsegmented
    - Strobila: 3000 to 4000 proglottids (Immature, mature, and gravid).
  - **Eggs:**
    - Operculated and small knob at the ends
    - Embryo: Hexacanthembryo (oncosphere).
  - **Larval stages:**
    - 1st Stage: Coracidium
    - 2nd Stage: Procercoid
    - 3rd Stage: Plerocercoid.

Life Cycle

- Definitive host: Man, dog, cat
- First intermediate host: Cyclops
- Second intermediate host: Fresh water fish
- Infective stage: 3rd Stage (plerocercoid) larva.

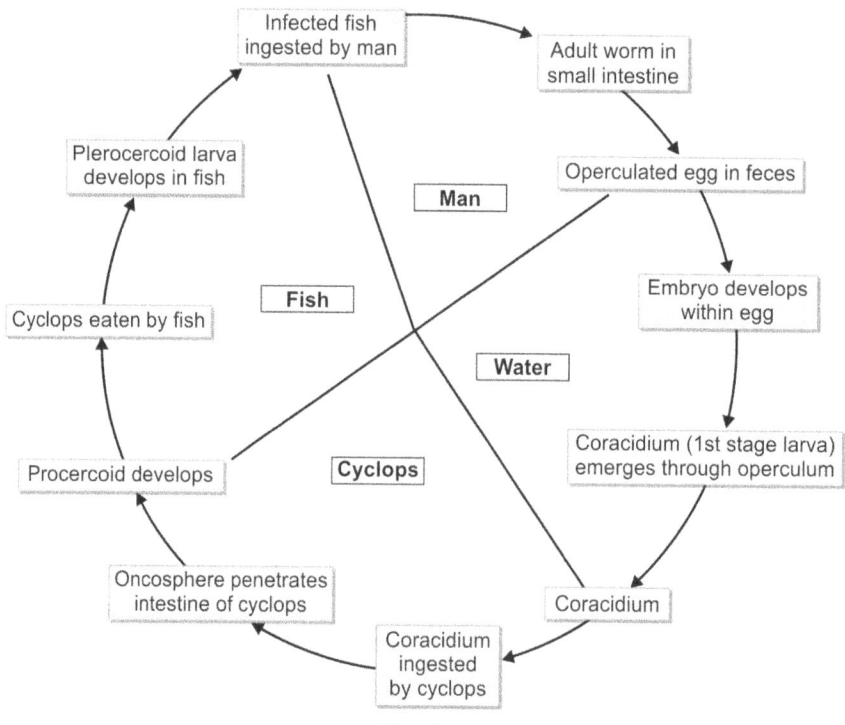

Fig. 48.2

Pathogenicity and Clinical Features

- Diphyllobothriasis: Sometimes asymptomatic
- Transient abdominal pain, diarrhea, nausea
- Weakness
- Pernicious anemia: 'Bothriocephalus anemia' due to deficient Vit B_{12} deficiency that leads to neurologic sequelae.

Lab Diagnosis

1. Stool microscopy: For detecting
   - Operculated eggs
   - Proglottids.
2. Serodiagnosis
3. Coproantigen test.

Treatment

Praziquantel and Vit B_{12} (if required).

Prophylaxis

- Proper cooking of fish
- Prevention of fecal contamination of natural water.

49 Nematodes

LARVA MIGRANS

- When larvae appear to lose their way and wander around aimlessly is known as larva migrans
  Seen in: 1. Non-human species of nematodes
          2. When infect immune persons
- Two types: 1. Cutaneous larva migrans   2. Visceral larva migrans.

CUTANEOUS LARVA MIGRANS (CREEPING ERUPTION/GROUND ITCH)

Etiology:
- Zoophilic nematodes:
  — Ancylostoma braziliense
  — Ancylostoma canium
  — Gnathostoma spinigerum
- Human nematodes:
  — Strongyloides stercolaris
  — Loa loa
  — Necator americanus
- Human trematodes:
  — Fasciola
  — Paragonimus
- Nonhelminthic: Flies of Hypoderma and gastrophilus.

Pathogenesis

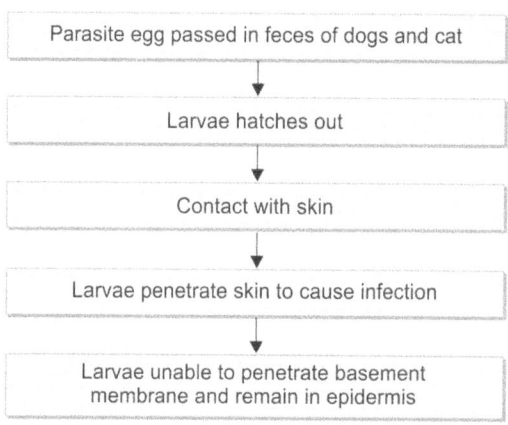

Clinical Features

- Itching papules develop into serpigenous tunnels
- Sometimes Loeffler's syndrome (refer ascariasis) may occur
- Rapidly moving lesion: Larva currens (S.stercolaris).

Diagnosis

- Based mainly on clinical features
- No eosinophilia (present only in Loeffler's syndrome)
- Larvae rarely seen in biopsy.

VISCERAL LARVA MIGRANS

- Infection by oral route
- Etiology:
    - Zoophilic nematode: Toxocaracanis, Toxocaracatis
    - Nonhuman nematode: Dirofilaria immitis
    - Human nematode: Ascaris lumbricoides, Strongyloides strecolaris.

Pathogenesis

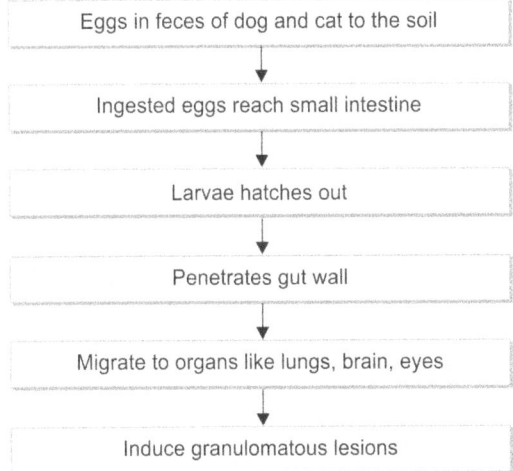

Clinical Features

- Most common in children
- Fever, hepatomegaly, pneumonitis, pica
- Neural larva migrans, ophthalmic larva migrans
- Eosinophilia.

Diagnosis

- Biopsy: Histological features of larvae
- Serological tests: ELISA, passive agglutination test.

Treatment

- DEC, Thiabendazole

Habitat	Nematodes
1. Small intestine	A.lumbricoides, Ancylostoma duodenale, Necator americanus, Trichinella, Strongyloides
2. Large intestine	Trichuris trichuria, Enterobius
3. Lymphatics	B.malayi, W. bancrofti
4. Skin/subcutaneous tissue	Loa loa, Onchocerca volvulus, Dracunculus
5. Mesentry	Mansonella ozzardi, Mansonella perstans
6. Conjunctiva	Loa loa

■ TRICHINELLA SPIRALIS (TRICHINA WORM)

Morphology
- Adult worms: Smaller nematodes
- Anterior half: Thin and pointed
- Posterior half: Clasping papillae (pair in male only)
- Larvae: Larvae encysted in skeletal muscle fibers
- Larvae is coiled: Hence spiralis.

Life Cycle
- Single host (definitive and intermediate)
- But 2 hosts are needed for preservation of species
- Mode of infection: By eating encysted larvae in pigs muscles
- Infective agent: Larvae.

Pathogenicity and Clinical Features
Disease is called Trichinosis
May be asymptomatic (commonly) or fatal illness (rarely).

Diagnosis
- **Direct Method**
  — Muscle biopsy
  — Stool examination
  — Xenodiagnosis (Rats are fed with meat and killed after a month to see larvae)
- **Indirect Method**
  — History
  — Blood examination
  — Serology
  — Bachman intradermal test
  — Radiological examination
  — PCR

Treatment
- Mild cases: Supportive treatment
- Moderate cases: Albendazole 400 mg BD for 8 days
- Severe cases: Glucocorticoids along with above.

Prophylaxis

- Proper cooking of meat before eating it.

DRANCUNCULUS MEDINENSIS (GUINEA WORM)

Morphology

Adult worm: Long, cylindrical smooth worm have a milky white cuticle
Viviparous
Larva: Broad anterior end and slender tail
Cuticle has striations

Life Cycle

- Definitive host: Man
- Intermediate host: Cyclops
- Infective form: Third stage larva

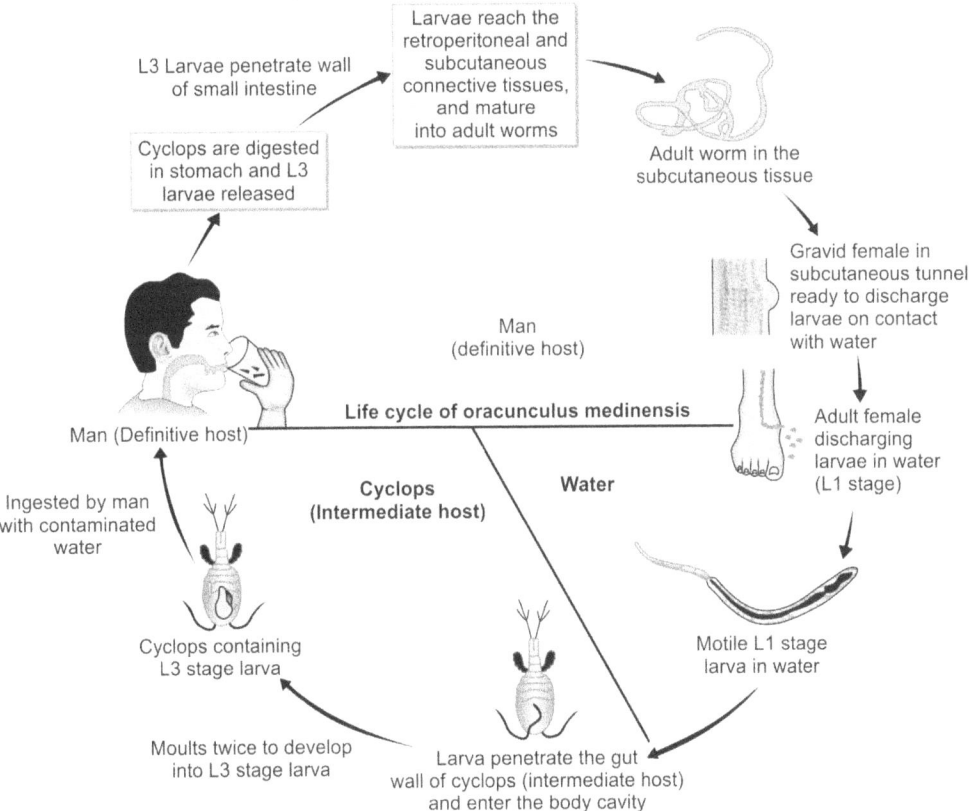

Fig. 49.1: Life cycle of dracunculus medinensis

Pathogenicity

- Causes Dracunculiasis/Dracunculosis
- Manifests when gravid female comes to lie under skin

- Body fluid of adult worm is toxic and form blisters
- Nausea, vomiting, pruritis and rash-before blister formation lasts usually 1–3 months
- Common sites: Between metatarsal bones or on ankles
- Sterile yellowish fluid in the blister with polymorphs, eosinophils, mononuclear cells.

Lab diagnosis
- Detection of adult worm from ulcer
- Detection of larva
- X-ray
- Skin test
- Serology (ELISA, IFA)
- Blood test (Eosinophil).

Treatment
- Antihistamines
- Metronidazole, Nitridazole, Thiabendazole
- Best method of worm removal is hoisting it around a stick
- Surgical removal.

Prophylaxis
- Boil water before drinking
- Destroy cyclops in water by chemical treatment with abate.

ECHINOCOCCUS GRANULOSUS (DOG TAPEWORM)

Morphology
Adult worm:
- Egg: Ovoid in shape
- Brown in color
- Hexacanth embryo
- **Larval form:** Seen in hydatid cyst.

Life Cycle
- Definitive host: Dog, wolf, jackal, fox
- Intermediate host: Sheep, cattle, man (accidental).

Pathogenesis
- Hydatid Cyst
  - Developed at the site of deposition
  - Three layers:
    1. Pericyst: Host inflammatory reaction with fibroblasts and mononuclear cells
    2. Ectocyst: Acellular, chitinous, laminated hyaline material
    3. Endocyst: Inner germinal layer

- A granular deposit (Hydatid sand) found at the bottom of cyst
- Fate of cyst: May be calcified
- Rupture into lungs or body cavity (dissemination).

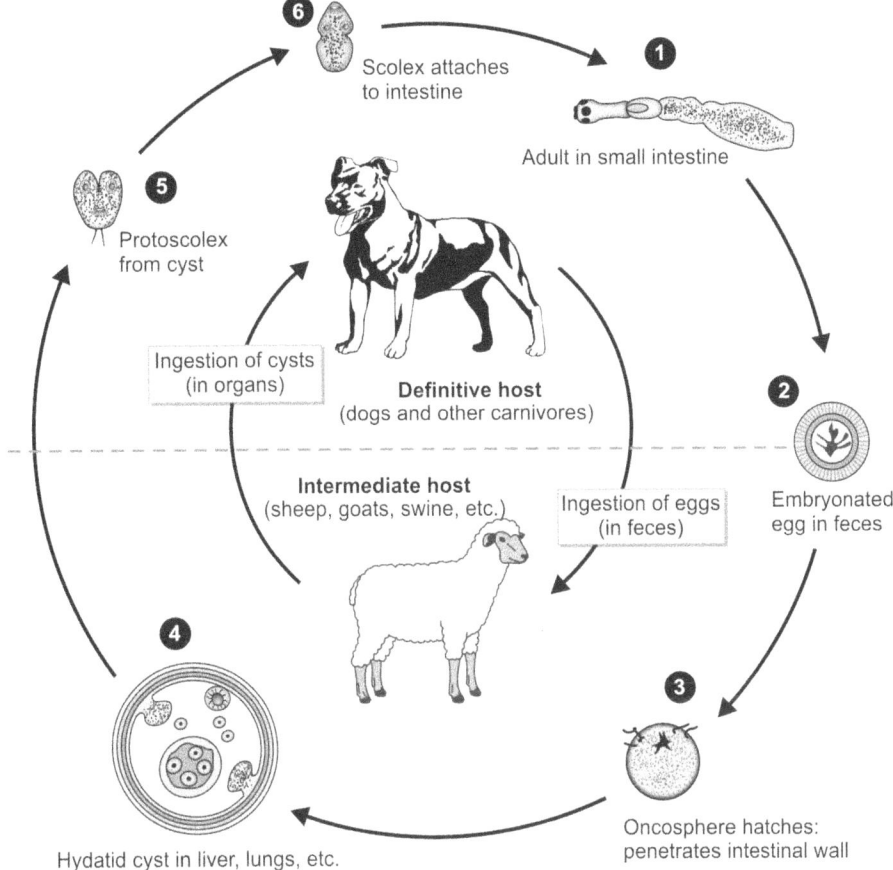

Fig. 49.2: Life cycle of echinococcus granulosus

Clinical Features

- Mostly asymptomatic and accidentally discovered
- Disease mainly due to pressure effects
- Sites:
  — Liver (63%): Hepatomegaly, pain, obstructive jaundice
  — Lung (25%): Cough, hemoptysis, chest pain
  — Kidney (2%): Pain, hematuria
  — Other: Spleen (1%), brain (1%), Bones (3%)
- Osseous hydatid cyst:
  — Formed inside bones
  — No laminated layer
  — So parasite erodes bony tissues by migrations.
- Brain: Epilepsy.
- Also by hypersensitivity, urticaria may occur and can cause fatal anaphylaxis.

Lab Diagnosis

Casoni's intradermal test

- Antigen collected from animal or human cysts and sterilized in seitz or membrane filters
- Method: 0.2 ml fluid injected intradermally in one arm Equal amount of saline injected as control on other arm
  Positive reaction: Large wheal of 5 cm diameter with projections in half hour 2° reaction: Edema and induration in 8 hours.
- Imaging:
  - USG: Water Lily sign
  - Procedure of choice
  - CT
  - MRI
  - IV Pyelogram
- Examination of cyst fluid: Scolices, brood capsules and hooklets
- Casoni's test (Immediate hypersensitivity test)
- Serodiagnosis:
  - Antibody detection: IHA, CFT, ELISA
  - Antigen detection: Double diffusion, CIED
- Others:
  - Blood shows eosinophilia
  - PCR

Treatment

- Ultrasound staging done and management depends on the stage
- Early stages: PAIR (Puncture, Aspiration, Injection, Respiration)
- Complicated cases: Surgery
- Chemotherapy: Albendazole, Praziquantel.

TAENIA SAGINATA (BEEF TAPEWORM)

Morphology

Adult worm:

- Scolex: Quadrate with suckers (Unarmed)
- Neck: Long and narrow
- Gravid segments: 4 times length compared to width

Eggs: Spherical

- Bile stained
- Hexacanth embryo

Larva: Called Cysticercus bovis

- Infective stage
- Seen as shiny white dots in infected beef (measly beef).

Life Cycle

- Definitive host: Man
- Intermediate host: Cattle (cow or buffalo)
- Infective host: Cysticercus bovis.

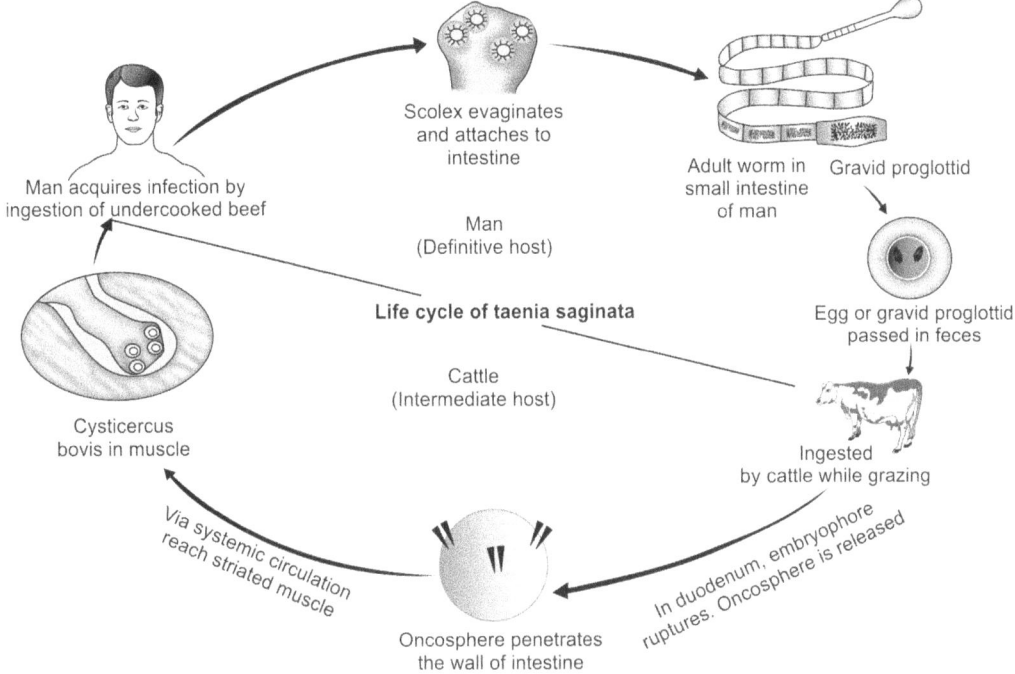

Fig. 49.3: Life cycle of taenia saginata

Pathogenicity

Intestinal taeniasis:
- Due to large size: Inconvenience in abdomen is felt
- Symptomatic cases: Vague abdominal pain, discomfort, nausea, diarrhea and weight loss.

Lab Diagnosis

Sample: Feces, blood
- Stool examination:
    - Eggs: Characteristic eggs of taenia
        - Formol ether sedimentation method
    - Proglottids: Species examination
    - Taenia antigen (Coproantigen)
- Serodiagnosis: Done by ELISA and IHA
- Molecular diagnosis: PCR.

Treatment

- DOC: Single dose of Praziquantel (10–20 mg/kg)
- Another drug: Niclosamide

Prophylaxis:
- Avoidance of eating raw and undercooked pork
- Maintenance of clean personal habits.

■ TAENIA SOLIUM (PORK TAPEWORM)

Morphology
Adult worm

- Scolex: 4 large cup like suckers
- Round rostellum with double rows of dagger shaped hooks
- Neck: Short and half the thickness of head
- Gravid segments: Same as T. saginata (except in table).

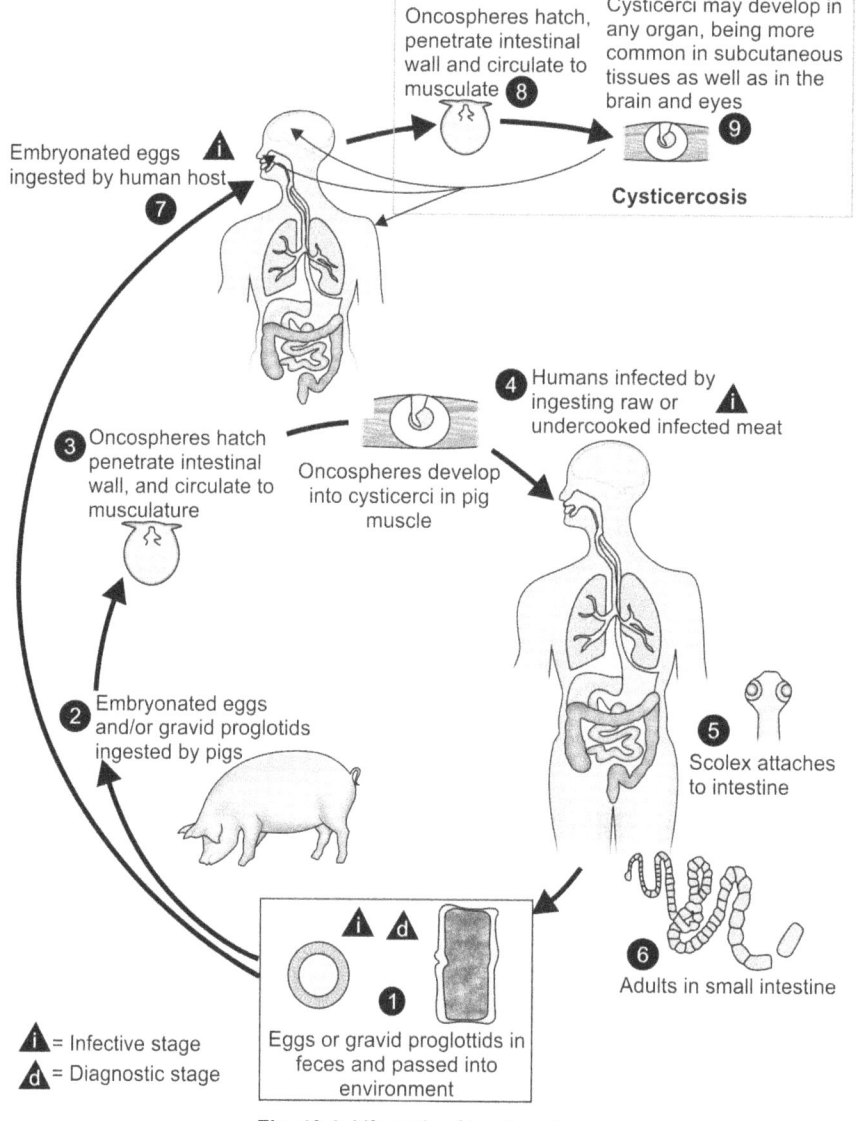

Fig. 49.4: Life cycle of taenia solium

Eggs:
- Spherical and bile stained
- Oncosphere embryo with 3 pairs of hooklets (Hexacanth embryo).

Larva:
- Called cysticercus cellulosae (Infective form)
- Contains single invaginated scolex (Bladder worm).

Life Cycle
- Definitive host: Man
- Intermediate host: Pig and man
- Infective form: Cysticercus cellulosae

Pathogenicity
- Intestinal teniasis (same as T. saginata)
- Cysticercosis: Any organ or tissue may be involved (common-muscle)
  Found in fibrous capsule (except in eye and ventricle)

Clinical Features
- Subcutaneous nodules: Asymptomatic
- Muscular cysticercosis: Acute myositis
- Neuro cysticercosis: Raised ICT, hydrocephalus
  Meningoencephalitis, paresis
- Ocular cysticercosis: Uveitis, iritis, conjunctivitis.

Lab Diagnosis
- Taeniasis (same as that of T. saginata)
- Cysticercosis:
  — Biopsy
  — Imaging methods: X-ray, CT scan, MRI
  — Serodiagnosis:
    – Antibody detection: ELISA
    – Antigen detection: ELISA

Taenia saginata	Taenia solium
Scolex: Quadrate, unarmed	Armed, globular
Proglottids: Expelled singly	Expelled passively in chains
Vagina: Present	Absent
Accessory Ovarian Lobe: Present	Absent
Testes: 300 to 400 follicles	150 to 200 follicles
Egg: Not infective to man	Infective to man
Uterus: 15 to 30 lateral branches	5 to 10 lateral branches

HYMENOLEPIS NANA (DWARF TAPEWORM)

- Smallest tapeworm
- Life cycle in one host.

Morphology

Adult worm

- Scolex: Suckers and hooklets seen
- Neck: Slender
- Strobila: With genital pores and gravid proglottids.

Eggs

- Inner embryophore with hexacanth oncosphere
- Non-bile stained

Life Cycle

Single host: Man

Clinical Features

- Most common in children: Asymptomatic
- Heavy infection: Nausea, abdominal pain, diarrhea
- Pruritis due to allergy.

Lab Diagnosis

- Demonstration of eggs in feces.

HOOKWORM

■ ANCYLOSTOMA DUODENALE

Habitat: Small intestine (mostly jejunum).

Morphology
- Stout, cylindrical worm
- Prominent buccal capsule
- Male worm smaller than females
- Copulatory bursa present in males and not in males EGG.

Oval or Elliptical
- Not bile stained, thin egg shell, a small gap between the ovum and egg shell
- Surrounded by transparent hyaline shell membrane
- Contains segmented ovum with 4 or 8 blastomeres.

Life Cycle
- Definitive host: Humans
- No intermediate host
- Infective form and mode of infection: Third stage filariform larva by penetration of skin
- Pathogenecity and clinical features:

- Larva
  - Ground itch
    - When filariform larva enter the skin
    - Severe itching
    - An erythematous rash develops which later becomes vesicular
  - Creeping eruption
    - Filariform larvae wander About the skin
    - Severe itching
    - More common with animal hookworm infection
  - Respiratory manifestation
    - When larvae break out of the pulmonary capillaries
    - Manifests as bronchitis and bronchopneumonia

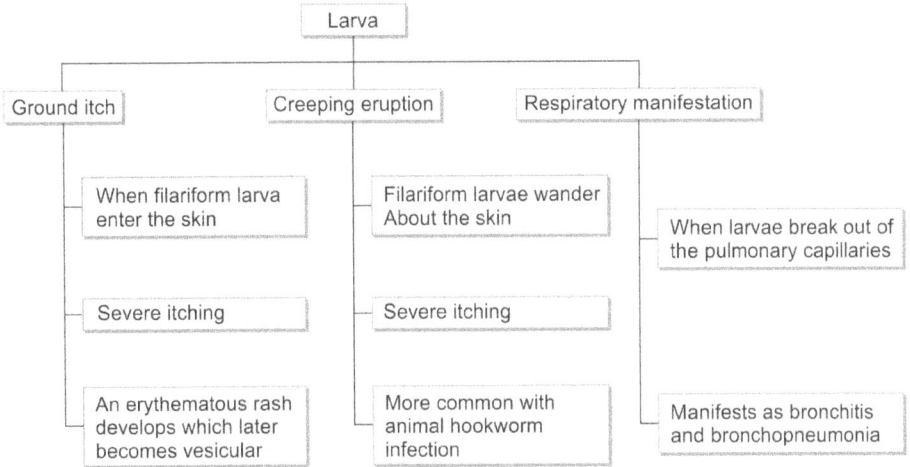

Adult Worm

Adult worm in human SI ⟶ sucks blood ⟶ microcytic hypochromic anemia with symptoms like exertional dyspnea, palpitation, edema, dizziness, epigastric pain, vomiting, dyspepsia.

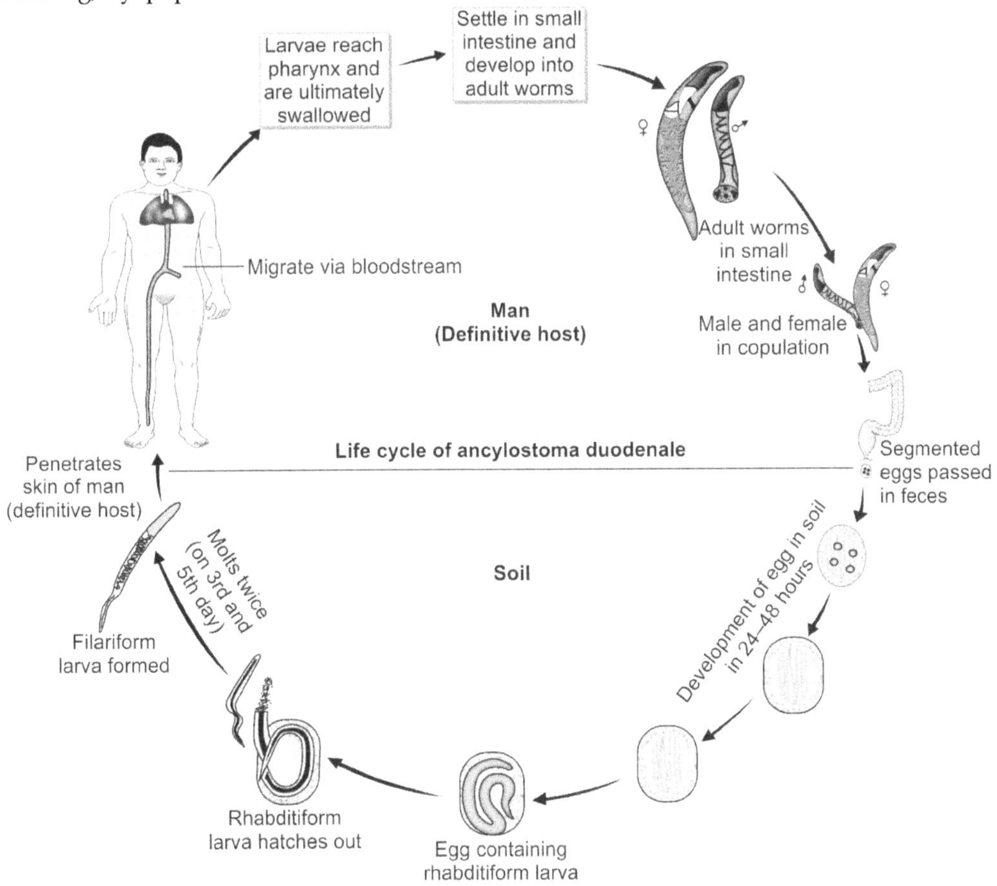

Fig. 49.5: Life cycle of ancylostoma duodenale

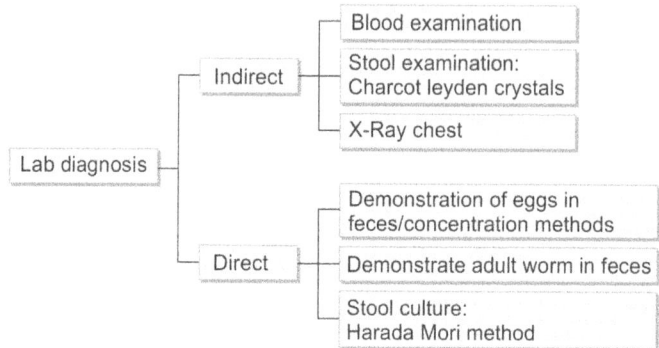

Treatment

Albendazole, pyrantelpamoate, correction of anemia.

Prophylaxis

- Prevent soil pollution with feces
- Use of foot wear
- Rx of patients and carriers.

■ NECATOR AMERICANUS

- Adult worms are smaller than A. duodenale

Difference between A. duodenale and N. americanus

A. duodenale	N. americanus
• Anterior curvature uniform	• Anterior curvature opposite to direction with body curvature of body curvature
• Buccal capsule with teeth	• Buccal capsule with semilunar cutting plates
• Vulva opens at junction of middle and posterior 1/3rds	• Opens little front of the middle

- **Pathogenesis, clinical features and lab diagnosis**: Similar to A. duodenale.

■ TRICHURIS TRICHIURA

Whip worm: Common name.

Habitat

Large intestine (cecum mainly)

Morphology

- Male worm is longer than females
- Male: Coiled posterior end
- Female: Very thin anterior portion.

Egg

- Bile stained
- Triple shell, barrel shaped
- Mucus plug at each pole and unsegmented ovum.

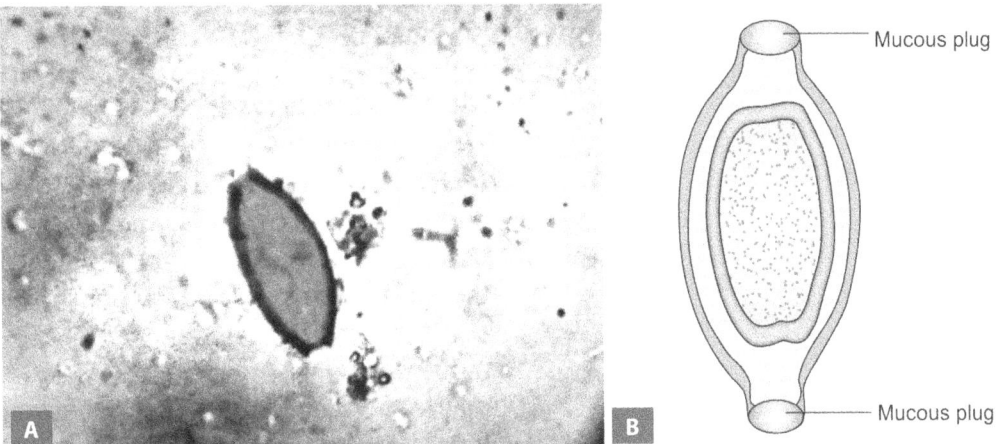

Figs 49.6 (A and B): Egg of Trichuris Trichiura: **A.** As seen under microscope, **B.** Schematic diagram

Life Cycle

- Natural host: Man
- No intermediate host
- Infective form and mode of infection: Egg containing rhabditiform larva by ingestion.

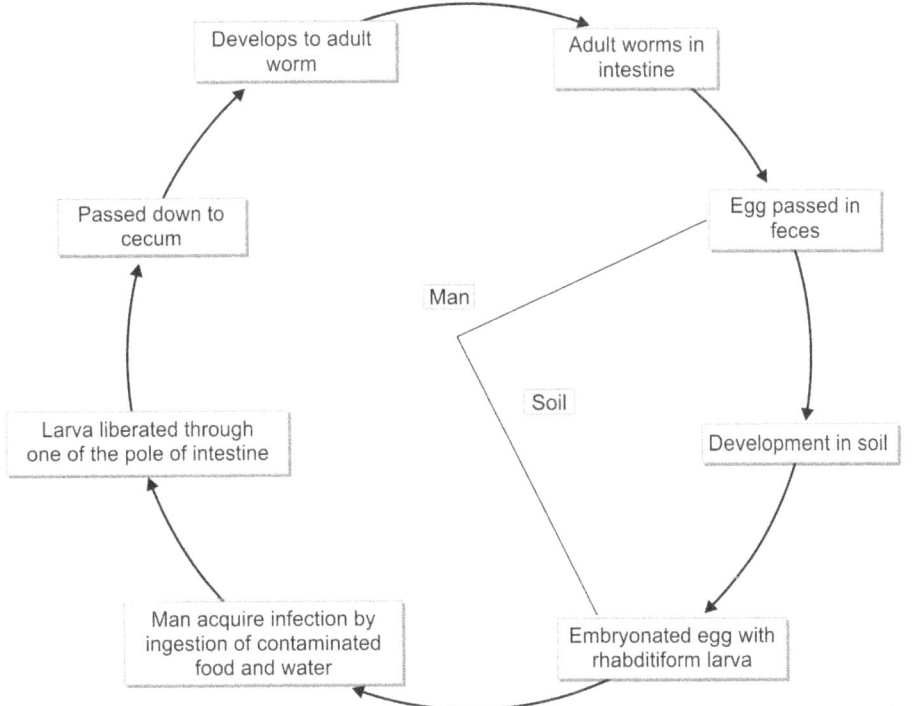

Fig. 49.7: Life cycle of trichuris trichiura

Pathogenicity and Clinical Features

- Trichuriasis
- Due to mechanical effects or allergic reaction
- Blood loss anemia and malnutrition
- Cause appendicitis.

Lab Diagnosis

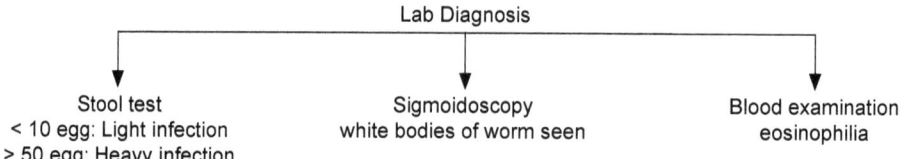

Lab Diagnosis		
Stool test < 10 egg: Light infection > 50 egg: Heavy infection	Sigmoidoscopy white bodies of worm seen	Blood examination eosinophilia

Treatment

Mebendazole or albendazole

Prophylaxis

- Proper washing of vegetables
- Avoid soil contamination of feces.

■ STRONGYLOIDES STERCORALIS

Habitat

Human small intestine: Duodenum and jejunum.

Morphology

Male Worm

- Shorter and broader than females
- Copulatory spicules
- Not seen in human infection.

Female Worm

- Thin, transparent
- Cylindrical esophagus
- Causes autoinfection.

EGGS

Larva formed immediately after eggs laid, larva seen in feces: No eggs in feces.

Larva

- Rhabditiform larva (L1 Stage)
  - Double bulb esophagus
  - Commonest form seen in feces.
- Filariform larva (L3 Stage)
  - Infective stage of parasite.

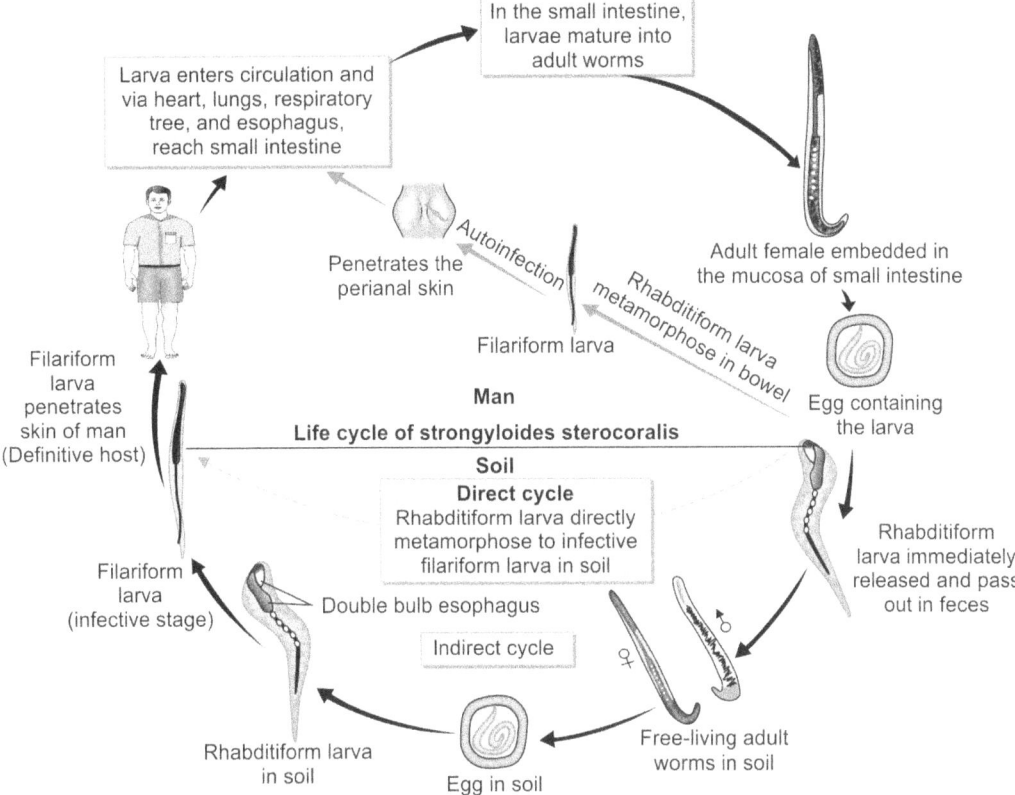

Fig. 49.8: Life cycle of Strongyloides stercoralis

Life Cycle

- Natural host: Man, dogs, cats
- Infective form: Third stage filariform larva
- Mode of infection: Skin penetration by filariform larva (L3 stage) and autoinfection.

Pathogenicity and Clinical Features
Cutaneous

Infective form ⟶ Filariform larva
penetrates skin and cause dermatitis, itching, erythema

- Larva currens: Rapidly progressing lesion by migrating larva

Pulmonary

- Larva breaks into alveoli from pulmonary capillaries
- Bronchopneumonia may be present which progress to chronic bronchitis
- Larva found in sputum of patient.

Intestinal

- Resembles peptic ulcer
- Mucus diarrhea
- Honeycomb mucosa
- Protein losing enteropathy, paralytic ileus.

Hyperinfection
- Immunocompromised
- Larva lodge in heart, lungs, brain, kidney, pancreas.

Lab Diagnosis
Microscopy
- Larva in freshly passed stools
- Concentration methods.

Serology:
CFT, ELISA, IHA.

Blood Examination:
Eosinophilia, raised IgE.

Treatment
Ivermectin.

Prophylaxis
- Prevent soil contamination with feces
- Use of footwear.

ASCARIS LUMBRICOIDES (ROUND WORM)

Habitat
Small intestine (mainly jejunum).

Morphology
- Cylindrical worms with tapering ends.
- Adult male worm: Smaller than female.

EGG
Bile stained:

Fertilized egg	Unfertilized egg
Round or oval	Elliptical
Covering of albuminous layer with rugosities	Do not form rugosities
Large unsegmented ovum	Small atrophied ovum

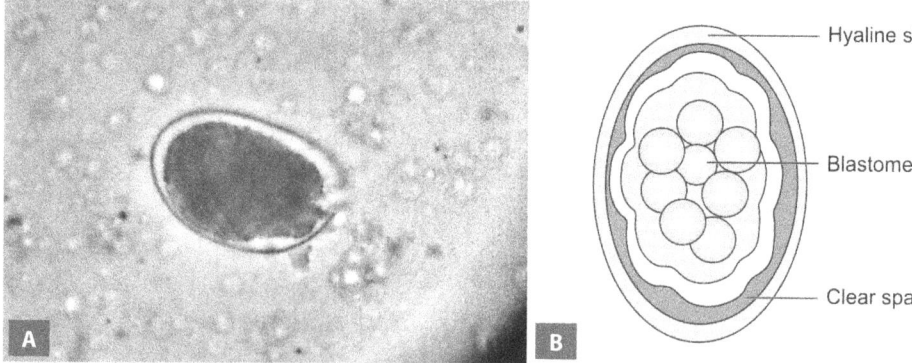

Figs 49.9 (A and B): Egg of Ancylostoma duodenale: **A.** As seen under microscope, **B.** Schematic diagram

Life Cycle

- Natural host: Man
- No intermediate form
- Infective form and mode of transmission: Eggs containing infective rhabditiform larva by ingestion.

Pathogenicity and Clinical Features

- Due to migrating larva
  - Allergic
  - Ascaris pneumonia: Low grade fever, dry cough, asthmatic wheezing, urticaria, eosinophilia, mottled lung infections.
  - Loeffler's syndrome: Charcot-leyden crystals in sputum and larva in gastric washings.
- Due to adult worm
  - Asymptomatic infection: Mildly infectious.
  - Pathological effects.
    - Nutritional – Protein energy malnutrition, vitamin A deficiency.
    - Hypersensitivity reactions to worm antigens.
    - Intestinal obstruction – Volvulus, intussusceptions.
    - Ectopic ascariasis.
      a. Wandering of worm.
      b. Acute biliary obstruction.
      c. Pancreatitis.
      d. Lung abscess.
      e. Appendicitis.

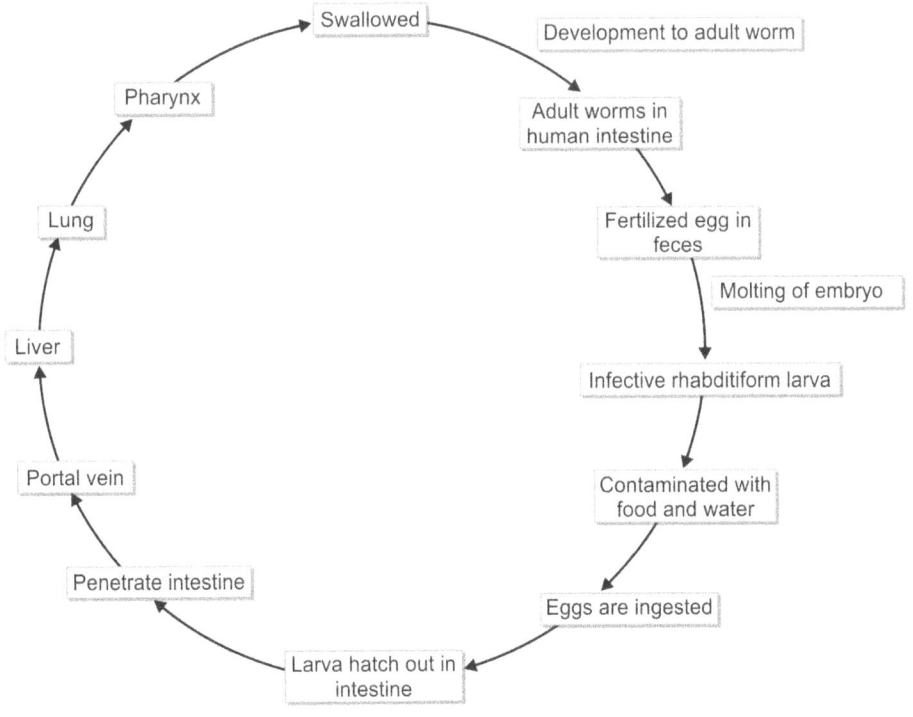

Fig. 49.10

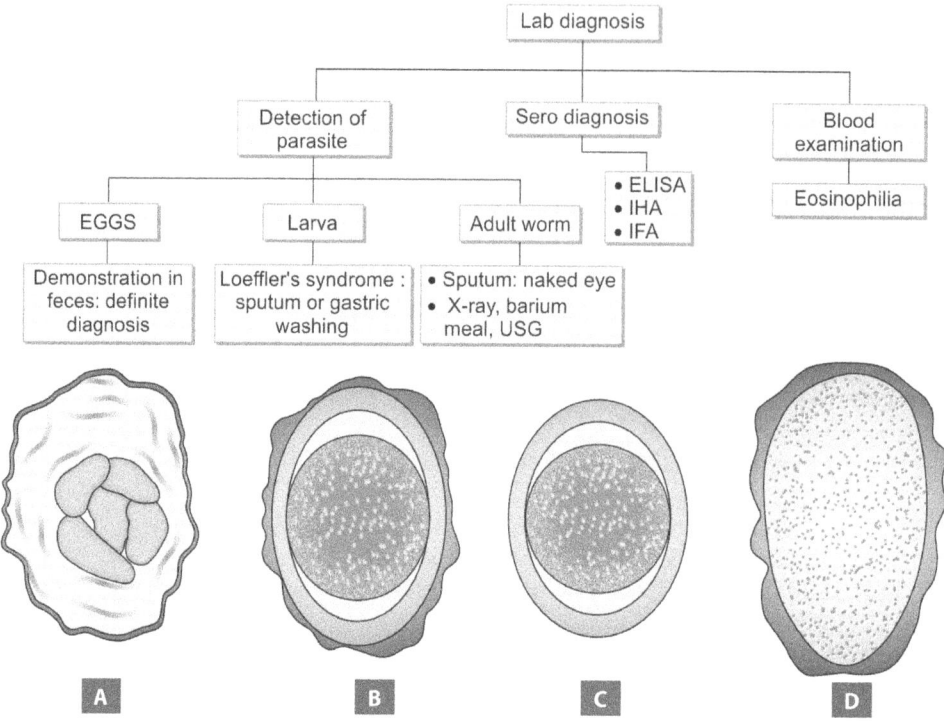

Figs 49.11 (A to D): Types of *Ascaris* eggs founds in stools: **A.** Fertilized egg surface focus, showing outer mamillary coat; **B.** Fertilized egg, median focus, showing unsegmented ovum surrounded by 3 layers of coats; **C.** Decorticated fertilized egg, the mamillary coat is absent; **D.** Unfertilized egg, elongated, with atrophic ovum

Treatment

Drugs

- Pyrantelpamoate: Safe in pregnancy
- Albendazole
- Ivermectin.

Prophylaxis

- Avoid eating of raw vegetables
- Personal hygiene
- Treatment of infected persons.

ENTEROBIUS VERMICULARIS (PIN WORM)

- Worlds most common parasite specially affects children
- Habitat: Adult worms: Cecum, apendix, colon

Morphology

Eggs

- Nonbile stained
- Planoconvex shape

- Thick transparent shell
- Tadpole shaped coiled larva.

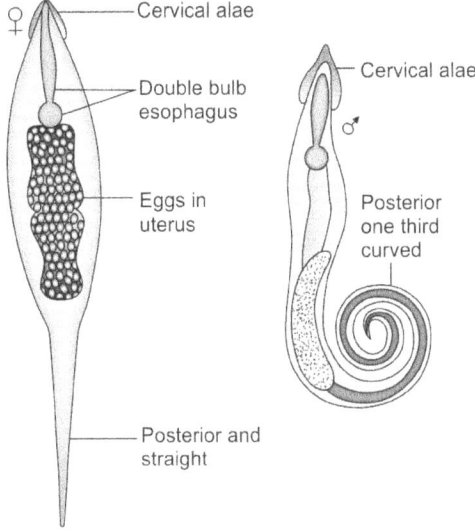

Fig. 49.12

Life Cycle
- Natural host: Man
- No intermediate host
- Infective form and mode of infection-ingestion of eggs through contaminated fingers or auto infection.

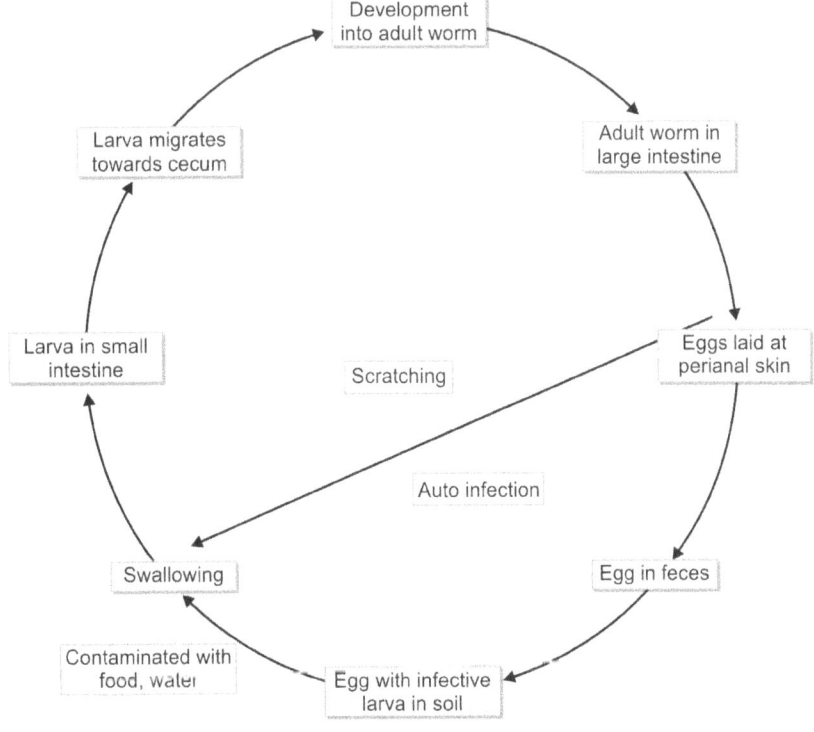

Fig. 49.13

Pathogenicity and Clinical Features

- Pruritus ani (pruritus of perianal skin): Occurs when it crawls out to lay eggs
- Nocturnal enuresis due to sleep disturbance
- Chronic salpingitis: Due to migration towards fallopian tube
- Appendicitis.

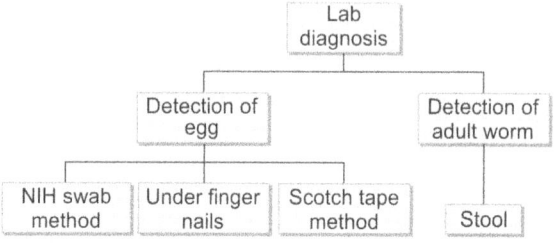

NIH Swab Method

- Cellophane part is used to collect specimen
- Microscope examination of cellophane part
- By spreading detached cellophane part over glass slide.

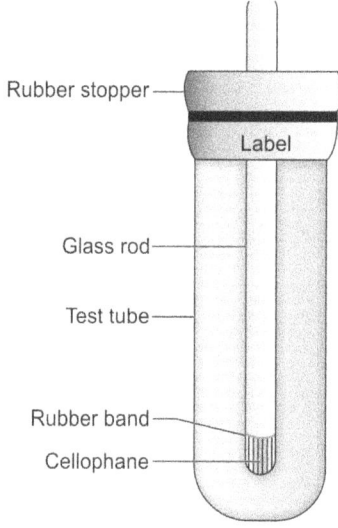

Fig. 49.14: NH swab. A piece of transparent cellophane is attached with rubber band to one end of a glass rod, which is fixed on a rubber stopper and kept in a wide test tube

Treatment

- Pyrantel pamoate
- Albendazole.

Prophylaxis

- Personal hygiene
- Washing of clothes
- Regular nail (hands) cutting.

FILARIAL WORMS

- Slender thread like worms
- Viviparous
- Larva is known as microfilaria.

Microfilariae

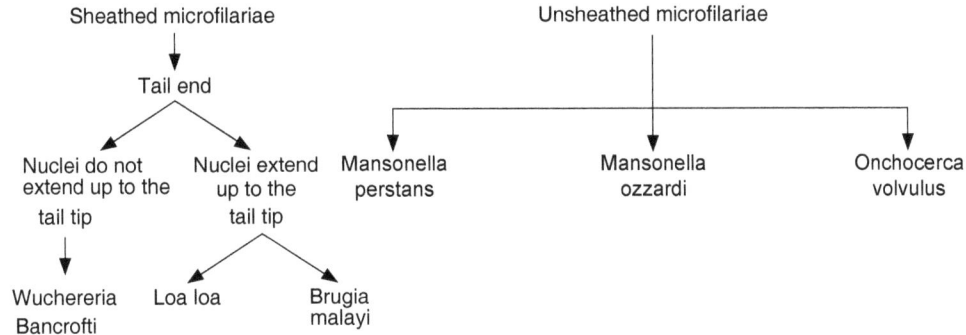

Nematode Infecting Humans

- Lymphatic filariasis
  - Wuchereria bancrofti
  - Brugia malayi
  - Brugia timori
- Subcutaneous filariasis
  - Loa loa
  - Onchocerca volvulus
- Serous cavity filariasis
  - Mansonella ozzardi
  - Mansonella perstans.

LYMPHATIC FILARIASIS

Wuchereria Bancrofti

Habitat
- Lymphatic system of man
- Microfilaria – blood.

Morphology
- Adult worm – Thread like worms
  - Tapering ends
  - Females larger than males.
- Microfilariae: Blunt head and pointed tail
- Covered by hyaline sheath.

Life Cycle

- Definitive host: Man
- Intermediate host: Female mosquito (India – culex)
- Infective form: 3rd stage filariform larvae
- Mode of transmission: Bite of mosquito carrying infective larvae
    1. Infiltrated with macrophages, eosinophils, lymphocytes and plasma cell
    2. Narrowing of lumen of vessels ⟶ lymph stasis ⟶ dilatation of lymph nodes
    3. Increased permeability of vessels ⟶ pitting edema
    4. Invasion of fibroblast ⟶ nonpitting edema.

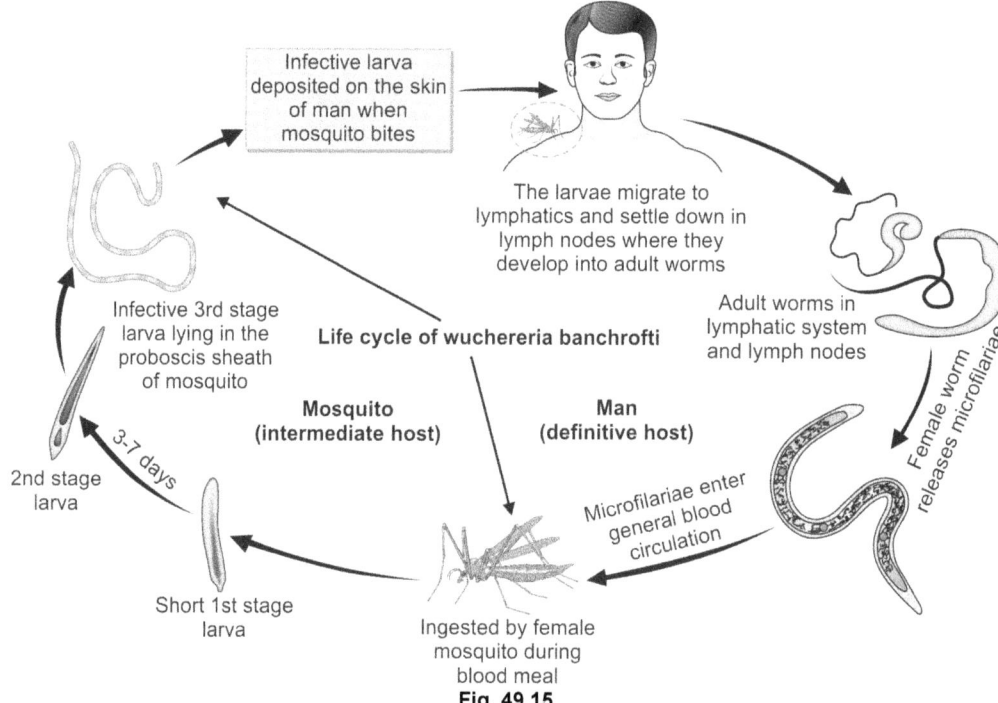

Fig. 49.15

Clinical Features

- Asymptomatic, acute adenolymphangitis and c/c lymphatic disease
- A/c adenolymphagitis fever
    - Lymphangitis: Inflammation of lymph vessels
    - Lymphadenitis: Inflammation of lymph nodes
    - Lymphedema: Initially pitting, later non becomes pitting
    - Lymphagiovarix: Dilatation of lymph vessels
- Hydrocele
- Lymphorrhagia
- Elephantiasis

Occult Filariasis

- Due to hypersensitivity reaction to microfilarial antigens
- Microfilaria not found in blood.

Clinical Features

- Eosinophilia (30–80%)
- Hepatosplenomegaly
- Pulmonary symptoms
- Classical features of filariasis absent.

Tropical Pulmonary Eosinophilia

- Manifestations of occult filariasis
- Low grade fever
- Dry nocturnal cough
- Loss of weight and pulmonary symptoms
- Marked increase in eosinophil count
- High level of serum IgE
- Chest X-ray: Mottled appearance
- Serological tests: Strongly positive.

Lab Diagnosis

Direct

- Detection of microfilaria:
  - Stained blood film: Thick and thin
  - Unstained film
  - Concentration methods
- Detection of adult worm:
  - Biopsy
  - X-ray
  - Ultrasound and Doppler.

Indirect

- Eosinophilia
- Elevated serum IgE.

Serology

- Antigen detection: ELISA
- Antibody detection: CFT, IHA, IFA.

Molecular

- PCR.

Treatment

- DEC is the drug of choice
- Given orally 6 mg/kg body weight for a period of 12 days
- Administration carried out in three ways

a. Mass therapy: Except for pregnant women, seriously ill patient and infants
b. Selective treatment: For those who are microfilaria positive
c. DEC medicated salt.
- Ivermectin
- Tetracyclins.

Prophylaxis

- Eradication of mosquitoes
- Detection and treatment of carriers.

LOA LOA

Morphology

Adult worm and sheathed microfilariae.

Microfilariae

Diurnal periodicity: Appear in peripheral circulation (12 noon to 2 pm)

Life Cycle

- Definitive host: Man
- Intermediate host: Chrysops Fly
- Infective form: 3rd stage of larva.

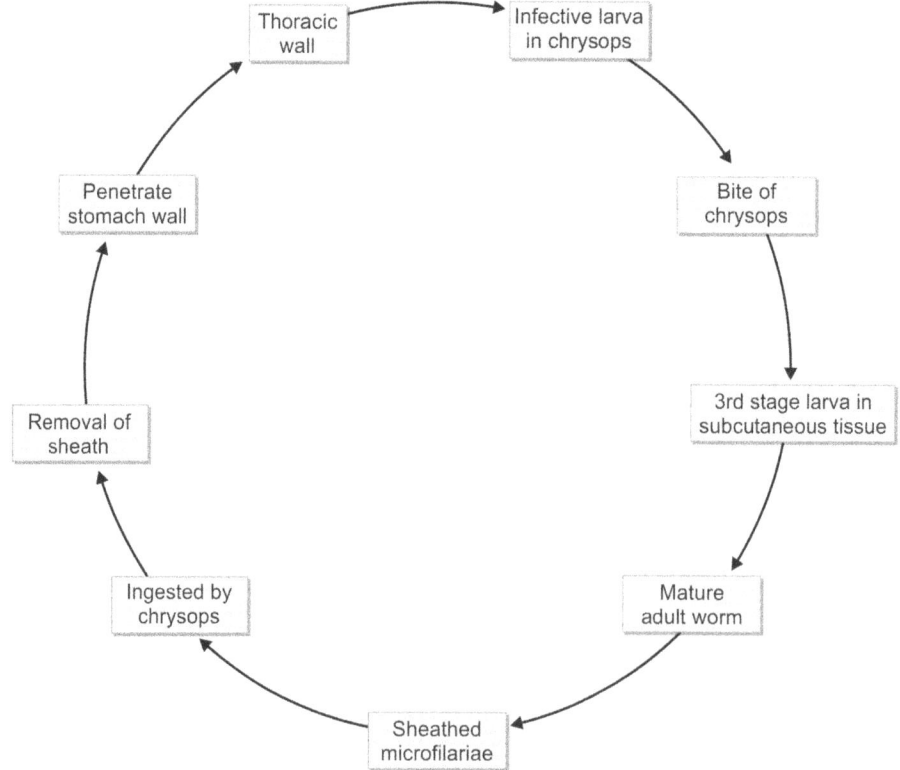

Pathogenicity and Clinical Features

- Calabar swellings or fugitive swelling: Temporary foci of inflammation due to wandering of larva
  Granulomata ←
  Ocular lesions ← painless eyelid edema
  Proptosis ←

Lab Diagnosis

- Detection of microfilariae or isolation of adult worm from eye
- Subcutaneous biopsy
- High eosinophil count.

Treatment

- Surgical removal of adult worms when they reach accessible sites
- DEC simultaneously corticosteroids given to minimize adverse reactions due to sudden death of large no. of microfilariae.

GNATHOSTOMA SPINIGERUM

- Causes larva migrans
- Zoonotic infection of man: Gnathosomiasis
- Eggs are oval brown with transparent knob at one end.

Life Cycle

- Definite host: Dog, cat, and other carnivores
- First intermediate host: Cyclops
- Second intermediate host: Fresh water fish and frog.

Clinical Features

- Migration of larva causes indurated nodule
- Also causes abscess and creeping eruption
- May reach brain or eyes causing damage.

Diagnosis

- Intradermal test: Using larval antigens
- Lesion biopsy.

Treatment

Albendazole, mebendazole.

50 Mycology

Morphological Classification
- **Yeast:**
  - Unicellular fungi. Example: Cryptococcus neoformans
  - Reproduce by budding
  - Macroscopy: Pasty colonies in culture
  - Microscopy: Round to oval forms.
- **Yeast like:**
  - Unicellular fungi
  - Reproduce by budding and fission. Example: Candida albicans
  - Macroscopy: Pasty colonies in culture
  - Microscopy: Spherical/oval forms in tissue and cultures
  - Filamentous (pseudohyphae) may be seen.
- **Filamentous fungi/moulds:**
  - Hyphae are either septate or aseptate
  - Hyphae may be of different shapes
  - Reproduction: Asexual means
  - Macroscopy: Cottony/woolly/velvety/granules
  - Microscopy: Thread like filamentous hyphae
  - Example: Aspergillus, Rhizopus, Mucor, Dermatophytes
  - Penicillium

  Mycelium of 2 types: 1. Vegetative
  2. Arial
- **Dimorphic fungi:**
- Grow as filamentous form in culture at 22–25°C
- As yeast form in cultures at 37°C and in tissues
- Example: Blastomyces, Coccidioides, Penicillium marneffi Histoplasma, Sporothrix schenkii.

Lab Diagnosis
- **Specimen:** Taken from affected site
  in c/o suspected disseminated infections, blood is to be collected.

- Microscopy: Morphology studied by
- KOH Preparation
  — Digest cells and other tissue materials
  — Enable fungal elements to be seen clearly
- Lactophenol Cotton blue (LCB)
- Calcoflour white (CFW)
- India ink preparation
- Methanamine silver stain and PAS
- **Culture**
  Media:
  — Specific – SDA
  — Nonspecific – BHIB, blood agar
  — Growth characteristics for identification
    - Rapidity of growth
    - Color and morphology
    - Pigmentation on the reverse
    - Morphology of hyphae

Teased Mount: Bit of fungal colony cut from culture
↓
Placed on drop of LPB Covered by a cover slip
↓
View under microscope
↓
Slide culture: To see the fungi with undisturbed morphology

Slide is placed in a bent glass rod in a petri dish
↓
1 cm 2 block of SDA is placed on slide
↓
Fungal stain to be identified is inoculated at four sides of agar block
↓
Block covered by a sterile cover slip
↓
Incubate at 25°C
↓
After 48 hours, growth appears
↓
Drop of LCB is placed on a fresh slide
↓
Cover slip is transferred from block of SDA into slide
↓
View under microscopy

Cellophane Tape Mount

Serology

(i) **Antibody detection:**
- Agglutination
- CFT
- Immunodiffusion

(ii) **Immunohistochemistry**

(iii) **Skin test**

(iv) **Antigen detection**
Latex agglutination

Classification of Mycoses

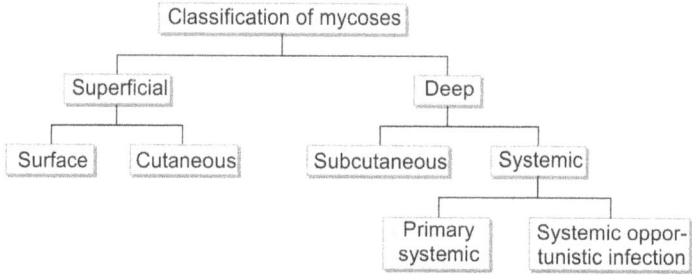

51 Superficial Mycoses

SURFACE INFECTIONS

- Fungi live exclusively on dead layers of skin
- No inflammatory response, only cosmetic effects.

Pityriasis Versicolor–Causative agent: Malassezia furfur (Pityrosporum orbiculare)

- Chronic involvement of statum corneum
- Asymptomatic.

Causative Agent

- Lipophilic yeast like fungus
- Malassezia furfur (Pityrosporum orbiculare).

Clinical Features

- Produce discrete, confluent macular areas of depigmentation
- On skin, chest, abdomen, upper limbs and back
- Its an opportunistic infections.

Diagnosis

- Sample: Skin scrapings
- Microscopy: abundant yeast like cells, short branched filaments
- Culture: Sabouraud's agar covered with olive oil.

Tinea Nigra

- Localized infection of stratum corneum (on palms)
- Black or brownish macular lesions.

Causative Agent

- Exophiala werneckii
- Exophiala catellani

Diagonosis

- Sample: Skin scrapings
- Microscopy: Brownish, branched, septate hyphae and Budding cells
  Culture: Grey/Black colonies on SDA.

PIEDRA

- Fungal infection of hair
- Firm, irregular nodules on hair shaft
- Nodules: Fungal elements cemented together on hair
- Causative agent: Black piedra, e.g. Piedraia hortae
  White piedra, Trichosporon beigelii.

CUTANEOUS MYCOSES

Dermatophytosis

- Infection of keratinized structures (skin, hair, nail) by keratophilic fungi called dermatophytes.
- May be acute or chronic.
- Twice as common in males as in females.

Causative Agents

- Microsporum (M. gypseum, M. canis, M. nanum) – affects skin and hair
- Trichophyton (T. rubrum, T. verrucosum) – affects skin hair and nail
- Epidermophyton (E. floccosum) – affects skin and nail

Pathogenesis

- Digests keratin by keratinases produced by fungi itself
- Pathological changes are due to fungi and their metabolic products.

Clinical Features

- Hair – Chronic type, forming crusts (Scutula) in hair follicles. Alopecia, scarring occurs.
- Kerion – Severe boggy lesions, Marked inflammation.
- Nails – Deformed, Discolored, Debris under nails. Friable nails.
- Skin – According to anatomic site
  (i) Tinea barbae – (Barber's itch) – bearded area of face and neck
  (ii) Tinea corporis – Smooth or non-hairy skin of body
  (iii) Tinea imbricata – Extensive concentric rings of papulosquamous scaly patches
  (iv) Tinea capitis – on scalp
  (v) Tinea pedis – of foot (Athlete's foot)
  (vi) Tinea manuum – involves hand
  (vii) Tinea unguium – involves nails
- Produce Circular, dry, erythematous, scaly and itchy lesions.

Lab Diagnosis

1. **Sample:**
   — Scrapings of skin and nail (from the edge of lesions)
   — Hair plucked from the scalp

2. **Direct microscopy:**
   — Wet preparation of specimen – scrapings in 10–20% KOH on slide for 10–20 minutes.
   — For nails additional time required (1-2 days)
   — Branching hyaline septate hyphae – positive for fungi.
   — In wet mounts of hair sample two types seen
   1. Ectothrix: Arthrospores seen surrounding hair shaft.
   2. Endothrix: Spores inside hair shaft.
3. **Culture:**
   — For species identification
   — Specimen inoculated into
   (i) Sabouraud glucose neopeptone agar + chloramphenicol (ii) Sabouraud agar + chloramphenicol + cycloheximide
   — Aerobically inoculated into plates – 21 days.

Macroscopy

- Trichophyton:
  — Powdery, velvety or waxy with pigmentation
  — Microsporum: Cotton like, velvety or powdery, white to brown
  — Epidermophyton: Powdery and greenish yellow.

Microscopy

- Trichophyton:
  — Abundant microconidia. (Scanty macroconidia)
  — Arranged in clusters.
  — Hyphae: Spiral, racquet, and favic chandeliers.

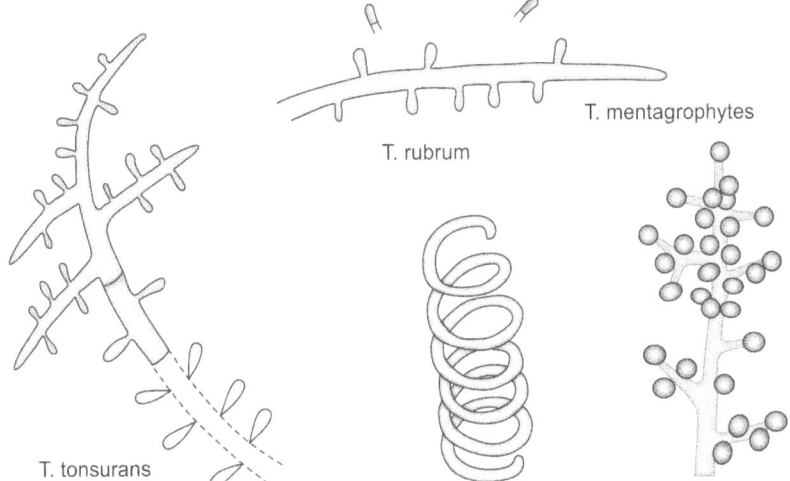

Fig. 51.1: Trichophyton species showing typical microconidia

Microsporum

- Microconidia scanty. (Predominant macroconidia)
- Large, multicellular, spindle shaped structures.

Epidermophyton

- Macroconidia: Multicellular, pear shaped in clusters.

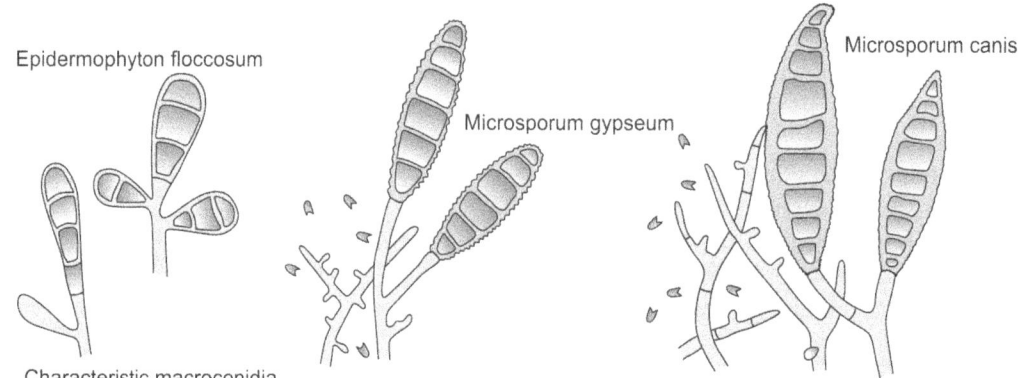

Fig. 51.2

Physiological tests
- Ability to penetrate skin
- Hydrolyse urea
- Hypersensitivity: Skin testing by fungal antigen – Trichophyton.

Treatment
- Topical preperations: Miconazole, Clotrimazole, Econazole.
- Oral preparations: Griseofulvin, Ketoconazole, Itraconazole, Terbinafine.
- Mild preparations: Topical imidazole, Whitfield's ointment.
- Severe infections: Oral Griseofulvin, Imidazole, Triazoles.

52 Deep Mycoses

SUBCUTANEOUS MYCOSES

Mycetoma
- Chronic, slowly progressive post traumatic infections of the subcutaneous tissue
- Site: Usually foot, may involve other parts.

Types and Causative Agent

1. Eumycetoma (Maduramycosis): Caused by fungi
   Example, Scedosporium, Madurellamycetomatis, Exophiala spp, Aspergillus spp, Fusarium spp.

2. Actinomycetoma – caused by Filamentous bacteria
   Example, Actinomadura, Streptomyces, Nocardia.

3. Botryomycosis – caused by Staph. aureus.

Pathogenesis

Minor trauma
Causative agent ↓
Subcutaneous swelling
↓
Enlarges in size
↓
Burrowing into deeper tissue
↓
Multiple sinuses in surface
↓
Seropurulent fluid with granules

- Granules (Grains) – Microcolonies of causative agent.

Diagnosis
- Demonstration of granules
- Color and consistency of granules: Vary with causative agent.

Brown to black	White to yellow	Red
• Madurella mycetomatis • Exophiala	• Nocardia • Actinomadura • Streptomyces • Scedosporium	• Actinomadura

- Actinomycotic mycetoma ⟶ Grains are composed of many thin filaments
- Mycotic mycetoma ⟶ Grains are broader and often shows septate and chlamydospores
- Culture, physiological tests and serology: Helps in diagnosis.

Treatment

- Treatment of eumycotic mycetoma: Vary with agents.
- Miconazole, Ketoconazole, Griseofulvin.
- Actinomycotic mycetoma: Dapsone, Sulfonamides, Clotrimazole.
- Amputation.

CHROMOMYCOSIS

Caused by dematiaceous fungi (pigmented).

Chromoblastomycosis

- Most common form of chromomycosis
- Seen in barefoot agricultural workers and wood cutters.

Causative agent

- Fonsecaea: Fonseceae pedrosoi
- Fonsaceae compacta
- Exophiala dermatitidis
- Cladophialophora

Pathogenesis and Clinical Features

- Trauma ⟶^(agent) enter the skin
- Warty cutaneous nodules – resemble florets of cauliflower
- Site: Feet and lower limbs.

Diagnosis

- Demonstration of sclerotic bodies in KOH mounts.
    - Sclerotic bodies ⟶ Round or irregular dark brown yeast like bodies with septa.
- Culture – SDA.

Treatment

- Amphotericin B
- 5-flurocytosine
- Voriconazole.

SPOROTRICHOSIS

- Chronic infection of cutaneous, subcutaneous and lymphatic tissue
- Seen in forest workers and manual laborers.

Causative agent
Dimorphic fungus: Sporothrix schenckii.

Pathogenesis and Clinical Features

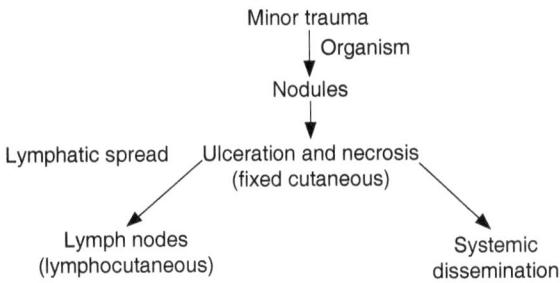

Lab Diagnosis
- **Specimens**
  — Pus, biopsy material, skin scrapings.
- **Microscopy (direct):**
  — KOH mounts of necrotic material
  — Asteroid body: Round or oval basophilic yeast like body.
- **Culture**
- Tissues and cultures at 37 °C: Yeast phase
- Mature and culture at 25 °C: Mycelia phase.
- **Serology**
  — In extracutaneous or systemic infection
  — Latex agglutination.
- **Skin test**
  Sporotrichin: Not used widely.

Treatment
- KI: cutaneous infection.
- Itraconazole: Lymphocutaneous.
- Amphotericin: Disseminated infection.

RHINOSPORIDIOSIS

- Chronic granulomatous disease.
- Development of friable polyps – nose, mouth or eye
  Rarely – genitalia, mucous membrane.

Causative agent

Rhinosporidium seeberi.

Pathogenesis and Clinical Features

- Mode of infection—not known
- Believed to be from stagnant water
- Polyps in nasal cavities, eye, skin and genitalia
- Hematogenous spread – rare.

Diagnosis

- Culture–not possible
- Histopathology ⟶ Spherules of 10–200 µm in diameter embedded in stroma of connective tissue and capillaries.

Treatment

Excision of polyp.

■ CRYPTOCOCCOSIS (TORULOSIS)

- Mainly caused by Cryptococcus neoformans
- Soil saprophyte seen abundant in feces of pigeons and other birds
- C. albicans and C. laurentii also cause human infection.

Pathogenesis and Clinical Features

- Infection acquired by inhalation, rarely through skin/mucosa.
- Pulmonary cryptococcosis: Lead to mild pneumonitis.
- Dissemination of infection: Lead to
  - Visceral: Simulate TB and cancer
    Bone and joints involved
  - Cutaneous: Varies from small
    Ulcers to large granulomata
  - Meningitis: Mimic TB/other meningitis
    Insidious onset
    Slow and progressive.

Lab Diagnosis

- **Specimen:** From lesion, CSF
- **Microscopy:** Indian ink stained wet film
  Budding yeast cells
  Capsules are prominent
- **Culture:**
  SDA : Smooth mucoid, creamey coloured colonies
  — Grow at 37 °C and hydrolyse urea
- **Animal inoculation:** Intracerebral/Intraperitoneal
- **Serology:** Demonstration of capsular antigen by precipitation

Treatment

- Amphotericin – B
- 5-fluorocytosine
- Imidazoles, triazoles
- Echinocandins.

BLASTOMYCOSIS

- Characterized by suppurative and granulomatous lesions in any part of body
- More chance for lungs and skin.
  Agent: Blastomyces dermatitidis.
  Source of infection: Soil.
  Mode of infection: Inhalation.

Clinical Features

- Primary infection of lung resemble TB or histoplasmosis
- Local: Cause focal/diffuse consolidation, miliary lesion or abscess
- Disseminated – spread from lung through blood steam and from multiple abscess
- Cutaneous – mainly on skin of face or other exposed parts
  — Initially papules around nodules develop and coalese to elevated ulcerative lesions.

Lab Diagnosis

Specimen: From lesion.
Microscopy:

- In tissue culture at 37 °C – budding yeast cells, double contoured wall.
- At room temperature – septate hyphae, conidia and chlamydospores also occur.

COCCIDIODOMYCOSIS

- Primary pulmonary infection
- Spectrum – Inapparent, benign, severe or fatal

Causative Agents

- Thermally dimorphic fungus
- Coccidiodes immitis.

Pathogenesis

- Through inhalation of dust with spores
- Asymptomatic respiratory infection.

Clinical Features

- Self-limited influenza like fever (desert rheumatism/valley fever).
- Less than 1%–c/c progressive disseminated disease. (Coccidiodal granuloma).

Lab diagnosis

- Dimorphic fungus
- Spherules in tissues and culture: 37 °C (With endospores).
- Culture (room temperature): Mycelial form: Also in soil.
- DNA probe on exoantigen testing: In biological safety cabinet.

Skin Test

DTH: Coccidiodin antigen.

HISTOPLASMOSIS

Intracellular infection of the reticuloendothelial system.

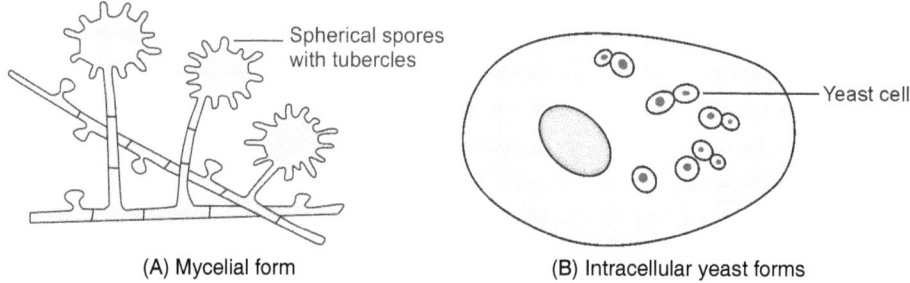

(A) Mycelial form　　　(B) Intracellular yeast forms

Figs 52.1 (A and B): H. capsulatum Mycelial and yeast forms

Causative Agent

- Histoplasma capsulatum
  - Histoplasma capsulatum. var capsulatum – Classical histoplasmosis.
  - Histoplasma capsulatum duboisii - African histoplasmosis.

Pathogenesis and Clinical Features

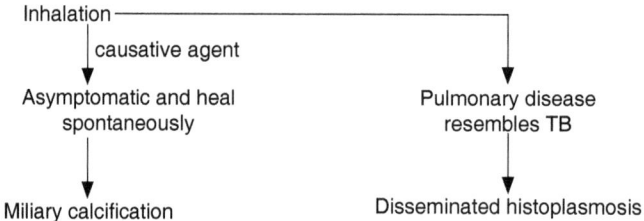

- Lymphadenopathy, hepatosplenomegaly, fever, and anemia.
- African histoplasmosis: Lungs are not commonly involved.
- Involves skin, s/c tissues and bones.

Lab Diagnosis

- Specimens: Blood, bone marrow, skin scrapings, biopsy of lymph node.
- Microscopy:
  - Classical histoplasmosis – Intracellular and extracellular yeast cells.
  - African histoplasmosis – Large thick walled yeast cells and giant cell formation.

- Culture – SDA
  - Yeast form: Tissues and culture at 37 °C.
    Oval budding cell.
  - Mycelial form: Culture at 25 °C
    White cottony growth
    Large thick walled spherical spores with tubercles (tubercular spores).
- **Serology:** CFT, Latex agglutination, Precipitation tests.
- **Skin test:** Using histoplasmin.
- **Treatment:** Amphotericin (DOC), ketoconazole, itraconazole.

CANDIDIASIS

Opportunistic infection mainly involving skin and mucous membrane.

Causative agent
Candida albicans.

Pathogenesis and Clinical Features

Cutaneous
- Intertriginous:
  - Groin, axilla, perineum.
  - Sharply demarcated erythematous lesions.
  - Paronychia and onychomycosis.
- **Mucosal lesions**
  - Vaginitis ⟶ Pregnancy.
  - Oral thrush ⟶ Bottle fed infants.
  - Intestinal candidiasis Sequale to excessive oral antibiotic therapy.

Complications
- Bronchopulmonary candidiasis.
- Systemic infections: Septicemia, endocarditis, meningitis.

Lab Diagnosis

Microscopy
- Wet film or gram stain
- Gram positive budding cell.

Culture
- On SDA and bacterial culture media.
- SDA: Creamy white, smooth colonies with yeasty odor
- Candida albicans differentiated from other candida species
  - Growth characteristics, sugar assimilation and fermentation tests
- Candida albicans: Chlamydospores on corn meal agar at 20 °C

- Reynolds: Braude phenomenon – Ability to form germ tubes within two hours when incubated in human serum at 37 °C.

Serology
- Agglutination detection
- Not helpful in diagnosis.

Skin Test

Treatment
- Amphotericin–B
- 5-fluorocytosine
- Imidazoles and Triazoles.

ASPERGILLOSIS

- An example of opportunistic mycoses
- Main pathogen is Aspergillus fumigates
- Other species are A. niger, A. flavus.

Pathogenesis and Clinical Features
- Causes a variety of clinical syndromes.
    - Allergic bronchopulmonary aspergillosis
        - Route on infection – inhalation.
        - Leads to hypersensitivity reactions. ⟶ Type I–atopic individuals.
          ⟶ Type III – Extrinsic alveolitis.
          ⟶ Combined Type I and Type III
- Fungus grows within lumen of bronchioles and get occluded.
    - Aspergilloma/Colonising aspergillosis
    - Fungal ball grows with pre-existing lung cavity.
    - Cavity formed by old TB or bronchiectasis.
    - Invasive aspergillosis
    - Fungus causes pneumonia ⟶ Dissemination ⟶ spread to other organs
    - Due to prolonged treatment with antibiotics, steroids, and cytotoxic drugs.
    - Superficial infection
    - Otomycosis, mycotic keratitis, nasal sinuses.

Lab Diagnosis

Specimen
- Exudate – Sputum.
- Tissue section – biopsy/postmortem material stained by PAS.

Culture
- SDA medium
- Velvety powdery colonies
    - A. fumigatus – dark green
    - A. niger – black
    - A. flavus – yellow to green.

Microscopy
- Stained by LPB
- Septate hyphae and bear conidia
- Conidiphores have swollen rounded end ⟶ Vesicles
- Spores formed in chains on elongated cells called sterigmata.

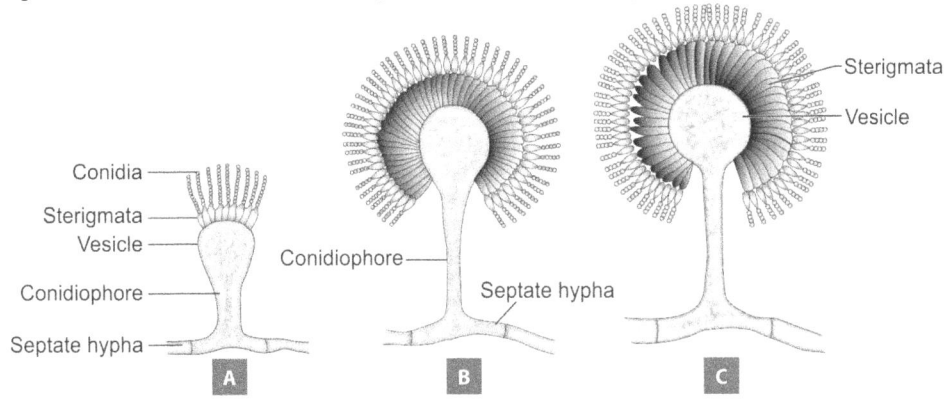

Figs 52.2 (A to C): Aspergillus spp: **A.** A. Fumigatus; **B.** A. Flavus and **C.** A. Niger

Serology
- CCIEP, ELISA, Immunoglobulin.

Skin test

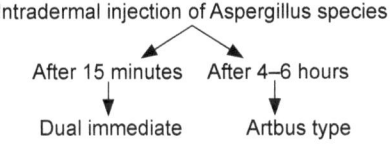

- Treatment : Amphotericin – B

PENICILLIOSIS

- Penicillium: Present in environment and grow on bread, fruits.

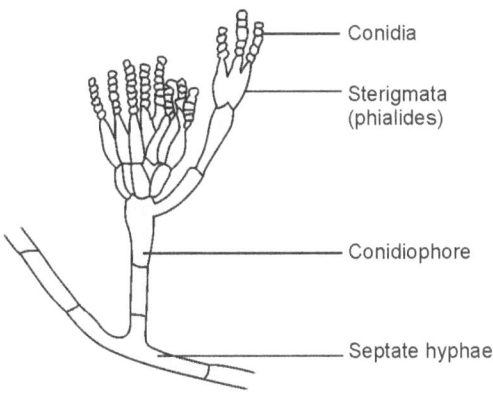

Fig. 52.3: Penicillium. Chains of conidia are produced by phialides, which are supported by branched conidiophores. Terminal conidium is oldest

Causative Agent
- P. marneffei (important opportunist pathogen).
- Dimorphic.

Pathogenesis and Clinical Features
- Disseminated infection.
- Multiple organ involvement.

Lab Diagnosis
- They are contaminants in culture media
  - Microscopy – Septate hyphae with branched conidia
  - Two rows of sterigmata bearing chains of spores.
- Macroscopy – Blue – green colonies.
  - Powdery surface
- Mycelia – red diffusible pigment.

Treatment
- Amphotericin – B followed by oral Itraconazole.

ZYGOMYCOSIS (MUCORMYCOSIS, PHYCOMYCOSIS)

Invasive disease caused by Zygomycetes.

Causative Agent
Rhizopus, Mucor, Absidia.

Pathogenesis and Clinical Features
- Primary focus is URT/nasal cavity
- Spores germinate and mycelia invades
- Orbit, Sinuses, Brain are involved
- In immunocompromised patients
- Diabetes mellitus – rhinocerebral form
- Lung – Primary site – Thrombosis and infarction

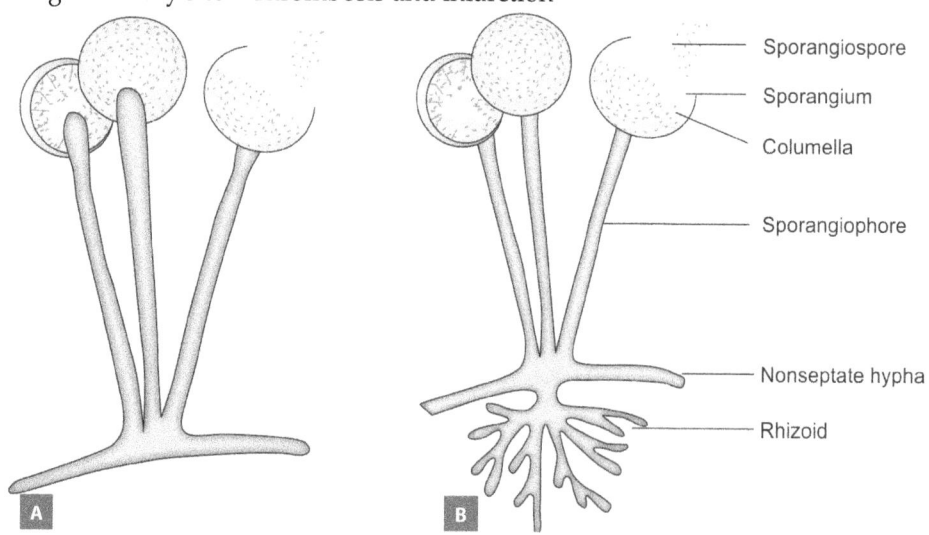

Figs 52.4 (A and B): Zygomycetes: A. Mucor, B. Rhizopus

Lab Diagnosis

- Specimen: Exudates – wet preparation with 10% KOH.
  Tissue: H and E preparation.
- **Culture:** On SDA without cyclohexidine.
    - Macroscopy – Grey white, cottony, fluffy surface.
    - Microscopy – Nonseptate broad hyphae.
    - Aerial sporangiophores end in a sporangium.
    - Mucor – branched sporangiophores and no rhizoids.
    - Rhizopus – has rhizoids and sporangiophores in groups.

Treatment

- IV Amphotericin – B + Surgical drainage.
- Diabetic control.

53 Otomycosis

Fungal infection of external ear.

Causative Agents

- Aspergillus niger
- Aspergillus fumigates
- Penicillium.

Symptoms

- Itching, pain and deafness.
- Secondary bacterial infection by Proteus and Pseudomonas.
- Leads to suppuration.

Lab diagnosis

- Same as that of aspergillus and penicillium.

■ OCULOMYCOSIS

Invasive infection of cornea – following corneal trauma.

Causative Agents

- Aspergillus species (A. fumigatus, A. flavus, A. niger).
- Fusarium.
- Alternaria, Aeremonium, Candida albicans.

Pathogenesis and Clinical Features

- Predisposing factors: Corneal injury and bacterial infection, use of corticosteroids.
- Fungal spores colonise injured tissue.
- Initiates inflammatory reaction: Hypopyon ulcer and endophthalmitis.

Lab Diagnosis

Specimen: Deep scrapings of corna collected under slit lamp microscope.

Treatment

- Local application - Amphotericin – B
- Nystatin
- Natamycin.

54 Mycotic Poisoning

Two types
1. Mycetism: Fungus is eaten itself.
2. Mycotoxicosis: Fungal toxins contaminated in food.

MYCETISM

- Example: Claviceps species: Ergot poisoning
  Coprine species: Coprine poisoning
  Inocybe species: Muscarine poisoning.

MYCOTOXICOSIS

Aflatoxin

- Produced by Aspergillus flavus – B1
- Aspergillus secretes aflatoxin – 'B_1, B_2, B_3, G_1 and G_2''.
- Present in ground nut, corn and peas.
- Cause hepatocellular carcinoma.
- Example: Fumonism – Fusarium species – Maize
  Orchratoxin – Aspergillus species – Cereals.
  Penicillium species – Bread.

Ergot Alkaloids

- Ergotoxicosis – Claviceps purpurea
- Fusarium – Trichothecenes
- Fusarium graminareum – Zearalenone.

APPENDICES

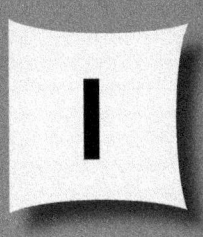

Appendix

Bacteria	Medium	Appearance
Staphylococcus aureus	• Blood agar • Ludlam's medium	• Oil paint appearance
Streptococcus pyogenus	• Blood agar • Pike's medium	• Mucoid colonies
Streptococcus pneumonia	• Blood agar	• Draughtsman or carom coin
Neisseria	• Mueller-hinton agar • Modified Thayer-Martin	• Weak hemolysis
C. Diphtheriae	• Loeffler's serum slope	• Clear or distinct yellow
B. anthracis	• Staining from cultures • Nutrient agar • Gelatin stab • Solid medium • Selective PLET medium • Staining with polychrome methylene blue	• Bamboo stick • Medusa head • Inverted fir tree • String of pearls • McFadyean's reaction
Cl. Tetani	• Gram staining	• Drum stick
Proteus	• Ordinary media	• Swarming
Shigella	• Selenite F broth • DCA/XLD	
Salmonella	• DCA/XLD • Wilson Blair • Selenite F and tetrathionate	• Black due to H_2S production
V. cholera	• VR medium and Cary Blair (transport medium) • Alkaline peptone water (enrichment) • TCBS	 • Yellow colonies
M. tuberculosis	• L J Medium	• Dry, rough, raised, irregular colonies with a wrinkled appearance
Leptospira	• EMJH media	
Mycoplasma	• PPLO broth	• Fried egg appearance
Legionella pneumophilia	• Buffered Charcoal Yeast Extract agar (BCYE)	

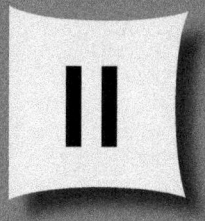

Appendix

VACCINES

Vaccine	Constituents	Dose	Route	Schedule	Contraindications
BCG	Live attenuated M.Bovis Danish 1331 strain	0.05 ml<4 weeks 0.1 ml >4 weeks	ID, above insertion of deltoid	Single dose, at birth	Immunodeficient children, pregnancy, generalize eczema, infective dermatosis
Hepatitis B	Subunit vaccine 1 ml cotain 20 microgram HBsAg	<10 years-0.5 ml >10 years-1 ml	IM, anterolateral aspect of thigh	0,1,6 months c/c dialysis-1,1,2,6 months	h/o allergic reaction to any vaccine component
OPV	Trivalent vaccine (type 1,2 and 3 viruses)	2 drops, as stated in the label	Orally	Zero dose at birth, 1st, 2nd and 3rd doses at 6, 10, 14 weeks booster dose at 16–18 months and 5 years	Immune compromised-leukemia, malignancy, on corticosteroids
DPT	D and T–toxoid P–whole cell vaccine	3 doses–0.5 ml	IM, anterolateral aspect of thigh	3 doses-6, 10, 14 weeks booster dose at 16-18 months and 5-6 years	Seriously ill children, children who had serious reaction to previous dose of DPT
TT	Toxoid adsorbed into Al salts	2 doses	IM	Booster immunization at 10 and 16 years, wound prophylaxis, 2 doses 1 month apart in pregnancy	Should not be administered after every injury if immunization is complete and last dose was received within last 10 year
MMR	Live attenuated Mumps virus Measles virus Rubella virus	0.5 ml	IM	Single dose,15–18 months	Pregnant women, patients on immunosuppressive therapy, severely ill patients

Contd...

Contd...

Vaccine	Constituents	Dose	Route	Schedule	Contraindications
Chickenpox	Live attenuated vaccine	0.5 ml	subcutaneously	Children– single dose 12-18 months, >12 years 2 doses 4-8 weeks apart	Immunocompromised persons, pregnant mothers
Pneumococcal vaccine	Unconjugated polysaccharide vaccine	0.5 ml	Subcutaneously or IM	3 doses 4 weeks apart, booster at 15–18 months	Anaphylaxis after previous dose
Hib vaccine	Capsular polyribosyl ribitol phosphate	0.5 ml – > 3 years, 0.25 ml – <3 years	IM or Subcutaneous	2 doses separated by an interval of 3 to 4 weeks	h/o allergic reaction to previous dose, children <6 months of age, moderate to severe illness

■ RABIES

Category	Type of contact	Type of exposure	Recommended postexposure prophylaxis
1	Touching or feeding of animals Licks on intact skin	None	None, if reliable case history is available
2	Nibbling of uncovered skin Minor scratches or abrasions without bleeding	Minor	Wound management Antirabies vaccine
3	Single or multiple transdermal bites or scratches, licks on broken skin Contamination of mucous membrane with saliva	Severe	Antirabies vaccine Anti rabies serum

■ POSTEXPOSURE PROPHYLAXIS

IM Schedule (Essen Schedule)

Five dose intramuscular regimen–The course for postexposure prophylaxis should consist of intramuscular administration of five injections on days 0, 3, 7, 14 and 28. The sixth injection (D90) should be considered as optional and should be given to those individuals who are immunologically deficient.

Site of inoculation: The deltoid region is ideal for the inoculation of these vaccines. Gluteal region is not recommended because the fat present in this region retards the absorption of antigen and hence impairs the generation of optimal immune response. In case of infants and young children anterolateral part of the thigh is the preferred.

ID Schedule

Regimen Updated Thai Red Cross Schedule (2-2-2-0-2). This involves injection of 0.1 ml of reconstituted vaccine per ID site and on two such ID sites per visit (one on each deltoid area, an inch above the insertion of deltoid muscle) on days 0, 3, 7 and 28. The day 0 is the day of first dose administration of IDRV and may not be the day of rabies exposure/animal bite.

Antirabies Immunoglobulin

Two types of RIGs are available: Equine Rabies Immunoglobulins (ERIG) and Human Rabies Immunoglobulins (HRIG).

Dose of rabies immunoglobulins: The dose of equine rabies immunoglobulins is 40 IU per kg body weight of patient and is given after testing for sensitivity, upto a maximum of 3000 IU infiltrated into and around the wounds. Remaining, if any, after all wounds have been infiltrated, should be administered by deep intramuscular injection.

Typhoid Vaccine

- Monovalent (S. typhi), bivalent (S. typhi, and S. paratyphi) and TAB (S. typhi, S. paratyphi A and S. paratyphi B)
- Nature of vaccine: Heat killed and phenol preserved vaccine
- Administration: Subcutaneous to outer aspect of upper arm
- Dosage: Adults and children > 10 years: 0.5 ml
    children < 10 years: 0.25 ml
- Schedule: 2 doses at 4–6 weeks interval
- Complication: Mild local reaction

Live Oral Vaccine

- Nature of vaccine: Live attenuated vaccine
- Content: Attenuated Ty2 Ia strain 109 organism per dose (enteric coated capsules of lyophilized vaccine)
- Administration: Oral (3 capsules)
- Schedule: A capsule on day 1, 3, and 5 one hour before meal
- Efficacy: Protection for 3 years
- Booster: 3 doses (day 1, 3, and 5) once in every 3 year.

New Typhoid Vaccine: Injectable (Typhim – VI)

- Content: Purified VI polysaccharide antigen of S. typhi Ty2 Ia strain (25 mcg per dose)
- Administration: Subcutaneous or intramuscular
- Schedule: Single injection
- Recommended only for above 5 years.

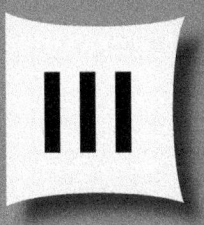

Appendix

GRAM STAINING

Aim

To study the morphology and Gram reaction of Bacteria.

Procedure

- Fix the smear by rapidly passing through the flame
- Cover the fixed smear with methyl violet for 1 minute
- Rapidly wash off the stain with clean water
- Cover the smear with Gram's iodine and keep it for 1 minute
- Wash off the iodine with clean water
- Decolorize rapidly with acetone. Hold the slide in a slanting position; add Acetone drop by drop (within 10 seconds) Wash immediately with water
- Counterstain with Dilute carbol fuschin for 30 seconds
- Wash off the stain with water
- Blot dry with filter paper wiping the back of the slide clean
- Examine under oil immersion objective. Open fully the condenser iris to admit maximum light.

Note

- Gram positive bacteria are those that resist decolourization and retain the primary stain, appearing violet.
- Gram negative bacteria are decolorized by organic solvents, take counter-stain and appear pink.

Mechanism

- Exact mechanism of Gram stain not known
- Gram staining is a property of intact cell wall and damage to cell wall will cause a Gram positive bacteria to appear gram negative
- Cell wall of gram positive bacteria contain thick peptidoglycan layer While Gram negative cell wall contain thin peptidoglycan layer and more lipids which dissolves on decolorization
- Acidic protoplasm of Gram positive bacteria binds the basic dye strongly and retains it

ZIEHL-NEELSEN STAINING

Aim
To determine acid fast bacilli in the given sputum smear and to grade the smear.

Procedure
- Fix the smear by rapidly passing through the flame
- Place the smear on a rack
- Flood the slide with Ziehl-Neelsen Stain (concentrated carbol fuschin)
- Wash off the stain with clean water
- Decolorize with 20% sulphuric acid until the smear is sufficiently decolorized, i.e. pale pink.
- Counter stain with Loeffler's Methylene Blue for 3–5 minutes
- Wash off with stain with water
- Wipe the back off the slide clean, and place the slide in a slanting position for the smear to air-dry
- DO NOT BLOT DRY
- Examine under oil immersion objective.

Principle
- Mycobacteria show the presence of coat made up of semipermeable unsaponified lipid material.
- This waxy lipid is made up of many complex fatty acids out of which —Mycolic acid is of great importance in staining reaction. This mycolic acid is present in the waxy lipid coat as a residue of peptide glycol lipid as well as in the cell wall as free molecules.

Mechanism
- Presence of mycolic acid in the cell wall
- Integrity of the cell wall.

IV Appendix

Q. P. Code: 205001   Reg. No......................

Second Professional MBBS Degree Examinations **(April 2013)**

Microbiology – Paper I

Time: 2 Hours   Total Marks: 40

Answer all questions
Draw diagrams wherever necessary

Essay: (10)
1. Read the clinical history and answer the following questions:
   A 20-year-old young male was admitted with history of fever with evening rise of temperature and cough since two months. Recently he developed hemoptysis. X-ray showed features of right lobe consolidation:
   – Mention the probable diagnosis and name the causative agent.
   – Describe briefly the methods of laboratory diagnosis.
   – What are the complications of the disease?
   – How the disease is treated?
   – What is the prophylaxis?   (2 + 4 + 1 + 1 + 2 = 10)

Short essay: (2 × 5 = 10)
2. Pathogenesis and lab diagnosis of syphilis.
3. Agglutination type of reaction in antigen-antibody combination.

Short notes: (10 × 2 = 20)
4. R plasmid.
5. Method of moist heat sterilization.
6. Enrichment media.
7. IgM.
8. Elek's test.
9. Prophylaxis of tetanus.
10. Wool sorter's disease.
11. Clostridium difficile.
12. Enterotoxigenic escherichia coli.
13. Chlamydial conjunctivitis.

Q. P. Code: 206001   Reg. No......................

Second Professional MBBS Degree Examinations (April 2013)
Microbiology–Paper II

Time: 2 Hours   **Total Marks: 40**

Answer all questions
Draw diagrams wherever necessary

Essay: (10)

1. Read the clinical history and answer the following questions:
   A 35–year–old man presented to the medical OPD with a history of intractable diarrhea for the past one week. He gave past history of multiple exposures six months back. On clinical examination he was emaciated and oral thrush was present.
   – What is the provisional diagnosis?
   – Mention the different routes of transmission in this condition.
   – Explain the pathogenesis of the above clinical condition.
   – Describe briefly the laboratory investigations.
   – What is the confirmatory test?
   – Mention any four important opportunistic infections associated with this disease.
   (1 + 1 + 2 + 3 + 1 + 2 = 10)

Short essay: (2 × 5 = 10)

2. Hydatid disease.
3. Pathogenesis and laboratory diagnosis of falciparum malaria.

Short notes: (10 × 2 = 20)

4. Giardiasis.
5. Cryptosporidium parvum.
6. Tinea versicolor.
7. Candida albicans.
8. Mycotoxins.
9. Mucormycosis
10. Infectious mononucleosis.
11. Prophylaxis of rabies.
12. Inclusion bodies.
13. MMR vaccine.

Q. P. Code: 205001   Reg. No......................

Second Professional MBBS Degree Supplementary Examinations **(September 2013)**

Microbiology–Paper I

Time: 2 Hours   **Total Marks: 40**

Answer all questions

Draw diagrams wherever necessary

Essay: (10)
1. Read the clinical history and answer the following questions:
   A 15 years old boy was admitted in ward with history of fever, malaise, anorexia and abdominal discomfort. He had a coated tongue, toxemia, relative bradycardia and splenomegaly on palpation of abdomen.
   – What is the probable diagnosis and name the etiological agent.
   – What is the pathogenesis.
   – What are the samples to be collected at different stages of the illness.
   – Describe briefly the laboratory diagnosis.
   – What is the prophylaxis.   (1 + 2 + 2 + 4 + 1 = 10)

Short essay: (2 × 5 = 10)
2. Pathogenesis and laboratory diagnosis of pulmonary tuberculosis.
3. Moist heat sterilization techniques.

Short notes: (10 × 2 = 20)
4. Eleke's gel precipitation test.
5. B-cells.
6. Bacterial spore.
7. Active immunity.
8. Bacterial conjugation.
9. Satellitism.
10. Toxic shock syndrome.
11. Listeria monocytogenes.
12. Bordetella pertussis.
13. 'Q' fever.

Q. P. Code: 206001 Reg. No.....................

Second Professional MBBS Degree Supplementary Examinations **(September 2013)**

Microbiology–Paper II

Time: 2 Hours **Total Marks: 40**

Answer all questions
Draw diagrams wherever necessary

Essay: (10)
1. Read the clinical history and answer the following questions:
   A 30 years old man presented with history of fever, chills on and off; O/E patient had hepatosplenomegaly, pallor++. A peripheral blood smear helped in the diagnosis.
   – What are the probable diagnosis and the etiologic agent?
   – Describe the life cycle of this agent.
   – How the disease is diagnosed in the laboratory?   (2 + 4 + 4 = 10)

Short essay: (2 × 5 = 10)
2. Life cycle of taenia solium.
3. Ebstein-Barr virus.

Short Notes: (10 × 2 = 20)
4. Laboratory confirmation of candida albicans.
5. Sporotrichosis.
6. Morphology of bacteriophage.
7. Coxsackieviruses.
8. Cytopathic effect (CPE).
9. Prions.
10. Gamma interferon.
11. Antigenic shift in influenza virus.
12. Chikungunya virus.
13. Negri bodies.

Q. P. Code: 205001   Reg. No......................

Second Professional MBBS Degree Examinations **(March 2014)**
Microbiology–Paper I

Time: 2 Hours   **Total Marks: 40**
Answer all questions
Draw diagrams wherever necessary

Essay: (10)
1. A 25 years old male comes to a medical outpatient department with complaints of high fever with relative bradycardia for the past one week, he has headache, coated tongue and hepatosplenomegaly. Answer the following:
   – What is the probable diagnosis.
   – What is the causative organism.
   – Describe the pathogenesis of this disease.
   – Discuss the laboratory diagnosis of this disease.
   – Discuss the vaccines used for prevention of this disease.   (1 + 1 + 3 + 3 + 2 = 10)

Short essay: (2 × 5 = 10)
2. Discuss about autoclave and its uses.
3. Discuss type I hypersensitivity reaction.

Short Notes: (10 × 2 = 20)
4. Louis Pasteur.
5. Lowenstein-Jensen medium.
6. Coagulase-test.
7. Bacteroides fragilis.
8. Satellitism.
9. Well-Felix reaction.
10. Natural killer cells.
11. Transduction.
12. Incineration.
13. Acinetobacter baumannii.

Q. P. Code: 206001 Reg. No......................

Second Professional MBBS Degree Examinations (March 2014)
Microbiology–Paper II

Time: 2 Hours Total Marks: 40
Answer all questions
Draw diagrams wherever necessary

Essay: (10)
1. Read the clinical history and answer the following questions:
   A one year old child presented with h/o inability to move the limbs associated with neck stiffness following a bout of fever. Immunization history was not available. O/E the child had flaccid paralysis.
   – What is the probable clinical diagnosis and name the etiologic agent?
   – Describe the pathogenesis of the disease.
   – How it is diagnosed in the lab and mention the prophylaxis available?
   (2 + 3 + 5 = 10)

Short essay: (2 × 5 = 10)
2. Life cycle of dracunculsis medinensis.
3. Dengue hemorrhage fever.

Short Notes: (10 × 2 = 20)
4. Otomycosis.
5. Cyst of giardia.
6. Acanthamoeba.
7. Intermediate and definitive host for toxoplasma gondii.
8. Hydatid cyst.
9. Egg of schistoma hematobium.
10. Eclipse phase in viral replication.
11. Significance of p24 antigen.
12. Enumerate enterically transmitted hepatitis viruses.
13. Cryptosporidium parvum.

Q. P. Code: 205001   Reg. No......................

Second Professional MBBS Degree Supplementary Examinations **(September 2014)**

Microbiology–Paper I

Time: 2 Hours   Total Marks: 40

Answer all questions
Draw diagrams wherever necessary

Essay: (10)

1. A 10 years old boy was admitted in pediatric ward with history of fever, toxemia and on examination. A white patch seen of fauces which bleeds on removal. He was not immunized properly. Answer the following:
   - Explain the probable diagnosis and name the causative agent.
   - Describe the laboratory diagnosis mentioning the methods of sample collection.
   - What are the complications of the disease.
   - How is the disease treated.
   - Describe the method of prophylaxis briefly. $(2 + 4 + 1 + 1 + 2 = 10)$

Short essay: $(2 \times 5 = 10)$

2. Pathogenesis and laboratory diagnosis of enteric fever.
3. Monoclonal antibodies and its application in clinical microbiology.

Short Notes: $(10 \times 2 = 20)$

4. Bacterial capsule.
5. Sterilization using dry heat.
6. Enrichment media with an example.
7. Toxic shock syndrome.
8. Differences between exotoxin and endotoxin.
9. Herd immunity.
10. Lyme disease.
11. Opsonization.
12. Differences between T' and B' lymphocytes.
13. Secretory IgA.

Q. P. Code: 206001　　　　　　　　　　　　　　　　　　　　Reg. No......................

Second Professional MBBS Degree Supplementary Examinations **(September 2014)**

Microbiology–Paper II

Time: 2 Hours　　　　　　　　　　　　　　　　　　　　**Total Marks: 40**

Answer all questions

Draw diagrams wherever necessary

Essay: (10)

1. A 45 years old male complaints of intermittent high grade fever which was cyclical and associated with rigor and chills. On examination he has hepatosplenomegaly. Answer the following:
   - What is the probable diagnosis.
   - List the species of organism which can cause this type of disease.
   - Discuss briefly the pathogenesis of the condition.
   - Discuss in detail the laboratory diagnosis of this disease.　　(1 + 2 + 3 + 4 = 10)

Short essay: (2 × 5 = 10)

2. Discuss the laboratory diagnosis of mycetoma.
3. Discuss the laboratory diagnosis of hepatitis B virus infection.

Short Notes: (10 × 2 = 20)

4. Rhinosporidiosis.
5. Naegleria fowleri.
6. Normal flora of skin.
7. Hydatid cyst.
8. Cryptosporidium.
9. Mycotoxins.
10. Dermatophytes.
11. Cutaneous larva migrans.
12. Papilloma virus.
13. Morphology of influenza virus.

Index

Page numbers followed by *f* refer to figure and *t* refer to table.

A

Acanthamoeba 151
   laboratory diagnosis 152
   life cycle 151
   morphology 151
   treatment 152
Acinetobacter baumanni 91
   pathogenicity 91
   treatment 91
Actinomycetes 90
Actinomycetes israelli 90
   clinical features 90, 91
   epidemiology 91
   laboratory diagnosis 90, 91
   pathogenicity 90
   preavention 91
   treatment 90, 91
Actinomycetoma 219
Acute glomerulonephritis 35
Acute rheumatic fever 35
Addison's disease 33
AFB staining 79
Aflatoxin 231
Agglutination reaction 25
Agglutinin 24
Agglutinogen 24
AIDS 143
   immunofluorescence test 144
   lab diagnosis 143
   line immune assays 144
   screening tests 144
   treatment 145
   western blot test 144
Ameba 147
   classification 147
   free living 147
   intestinal 147
Amebiasis
   lab diagnosis 149
Amebic liver abscess 150
   prophylaxis 150
   treatment 150
Aminoglycosides
   pseudomonas aeruginosa 73
Amoxicillin
   in *helicobacter pylori* 92

Anaerobic media 10
Ancylostoma duodenale 196
   clinical features 203
   life cycle 196
Anthrax 48
   cutaneous 48
      stages 48
   gastrointestinal 48
   pulmonary 48
   treatment 49
Anthrax toxin 47
Antibodies 20
Antigen antibody reaction 24
Antigenicity 20
Antigens 20
   biological classes of 20
   complete 20
   haptens 20
   T-cell dependent 20
   T-cell independent 20
Antirabies immunoglobulin 238
Arbovirus 121
Arthus type reactions 31
Ascaris lumbricoides 202
   life cycle 203
   prophylaxis 204
   treatment 204
Ascoli's thermoprecipitin test 49
Aspergillosis 226
   pathogenesis and clinical features 226
Atypical pneumonia 88
   lab diagnosis 88
   treatment 89
Autoclave 5
Autoimmune disease
   general features 33
Autoimmune hemolytic anemia 33
Autoimmune orchitis 33
Autoimmunity 33
   classification 33
   hemolytic 33
   localized 33
   mechanism of 33
   pathogenesis 33
   systemic 33

Azithromycin
    in Neisseria gonorrhea 44

B

Bacillary dysentery 60
    lab diagnosis 60
    treatment 61
Bacillus anthracis 47
    morphology 47
    pathogenicity 47
Bacteremia 17
Bacterial cell wall 16
Bacterial growth curve 2
    lag phase 3
    log (exponential) phase 3
    phase of decline 3
    stationary phase 3
Bacterial growth curve 3f
Bacterial spore 2, 2f
Bacteriophage 105
    life cycle 105
        lysogenic cycle 107
        lytic cycle 105
    morphology 105
Bacteroides fragilis 65
BCG 236
Benzathine penicillin
    in syphilis 85
Benzyl penicillin
    in staphylococcus infection 40
Biological false positive reactions (BFP) 84
Bird fancier's disease 100
Blastomycosis 223
Blood flukes 177
Bordetella pertussis 66
    clinical features 66
    complications 66
    epidemiology 66
    lab diagnosis 67
    treatment 67
    virulence factors 66
Borellia 65
Botryomycosis 219
Botulism 51
    clinical features 52
    forms of 52
    infant 52
    laboratory diagnosis 52
    pathogenecity 51
    wound 52
Brucella 74
Brucella melitensis 74
    laboratory diagnosis 74
    pathogenecity 74
    prophylaxis 75
    standard agglutination test 75
    treatment 75
Buffered glycerol saline 10
Burkholderia pseudomallei 73

C

Camp test 35
Candidiasis 225
Carrier 16
    chronic 16
    convalescent 16
    temporary 16
Ceftazidime
    in pseudomonas aeruginosa 73
Ceftriaxone
    in neisseria gonorrhea 44
    in syphilis 85
Cellophane tape mount 214
Cephalosporins
    in streptococcus pneumoniae 37
Cestodes 183
Chaga's disease 168
Chickenpox 111, 237
    complications 111
    in pregnancy 111
    lab diagnosis 111
    pathogenecity and clinical features 111
    prophylaxis 112
    treatment 112
Chikungunya 121
    clinical features 121
    lab diagnosis 121
    pathogenesis 121
Chlamydiae 98
    bacterial features 98
    morphology 98
    pathogenesis 99
    treatment 100
    viral features 98
Chlamydiae psittaci 98
Chlamydia pneumonia 100
    lab diagnosis 100
Chlamydia trachomatis 98
Chloroquine 166
Cholera 45
    clinical features 46
    lab diagnosis 46
    pathogenesis 45
    prophylaxis 46
    treatment 46
Cholera toxin 45

Chromoblastomycosis 220
    causative agent 220
    clinical features 220
    treatment 220
Chromomycosis 220
Ciprofloxacin
    in anthrax 49
    in Neisseria gonorrhea 44
    in Neisseria meningitidis 42
    Pseudomonas aeruginosa 73
Clarithromycin
    in *helicobacter pylori* 92
Classical rubella syndrome 134
Clostridium 50
    classification 50
Clostridium tetani 53
Coccidia 161
Coccidiodomycosis 223
Cold agglutination test 89
Cold sterilization 7
Complement fixation test 25, 26f
    indirect 26
Coomb's test 25
    and gell classification 29
    direct 25
    indirect 25
Coronaviruses 135
Corynebacterium diphtheria 70
    lab diagnosis 70
    pathogenicity 70
    tissue culture test 71
    toxin 70
Cotrimoxazole
    in Brucella melitensis 75
Coxsackie virus 139
    clinical features 139
Coxsackie virus A 137
Coxsackie virus B 137t
Cryptococcosis 222
    pathogenesis and clinical features 222
Cryptosporidium parvum 157
    cycle 157
    lab diagnosis 158
    life cycle 158
    morphology 157
    pathogenicity 158
    treatment 158
Culture media 8
    special media 8
Culture methods 10
    aerobic 10
    anaerobic 10
Cutaneous amebiasis 149
Cutaneous larva migrans 186
    diagnosis 187
    pathogenesis 186

Cutaneous mycoses 216
    causative agents 216
    clinical features 216
    lab diagnosis 216
Cyclophyllidea 183

D

Deep mycoses 219
Dengue fever 123
    clinical features 123
    lab diagnosis 123
Dermatophytosis 216
Desoxycholate citrate 9
Diarrhea 58
Differential media 9
Dimorphic fungi 212
Diphtheria bacilli 24
Diphyllobothrium latum 183, 184
    clinical features 185
    lab diagnosis 185
    life cycle 184
    treatment 185
Disinfection 4
Doxycyclin
    in anthrax 49
    in brucella melitensis 75
DPT 236
Dracunculus medinensis 189
    lab diagnosis 190
    life cycle 189
    pathogenicity 189
    treatment 190
Dreyer's tube 63
Drug resistance
    clinical significance 15
    mechanism 14
        in bacteria 15
Dry heat 4
Dwarf tapeworm 195

E

Echinococcus granulosus 190
    clinical features 191
    life cycle 190
    morphology 190
    pathogenesis 190
    treatment 192
Echovirus 137
Ectoparasite 146
Ehrlichia 95
Electroimmunodiffusion 25
Elek's gel precipitation test 71
ELISA *See* enzyme linked immune sorbent assay
Endemic 17

Endemic typhus 95
Endoparasites 146
Endotoxins 17
Enriched media 9
Enrichment media 9
Entamoeba histolytica 147
  life cycle 148
  morphology 147
Enteric fever 61
  carriers 61
  clinical features 61
  complications 61
  multidrug resistant 64
  pathogenesis 61
  prophylaxis 64
  treatment 64
Enteroaggregative E coli (EAEC) 59
Enterobacteriaceae 55
  classification 55
Enterobius vermicularis 204
  clinical features 206
  life cycle 205
  treatment 206
Enterohemorrhagic E coli (EHEC) 59
  lab diagnosis 59
  pathogenesis 59
Enteroinvasive E coli (EIEC) 58
  lab diagnosis 59
Enteropathogenic E coli (EPEC) 58
  pathogenesis 58
Enterotoxigenic E coli (ETEC) 58
  diagnosis 58
  pathogenesis 58
Enterovirus 137
Enzyme linked immune sorbent assay 27
  procedure 27
  types 27
  uses 27
Epidemic 17
Epidemic typhus 94
Epidermophyton 218
Epitope 20
Ergot alkaloids 231
Escherichia coli 55
  antigenic structure 55
  clinical features 56
  diarrheagenic 58
  enterotoxins 56
  virulence factors 55
Eubacterium 65
Eumycetoma 219
Exotoxins 17
Expanded rubella syndrome 134
Extraintestinal amebiasis 149

F

Fasciola hepatica 179
Fasciolopsis buski 175
  lab diagnosis 176
  life cycle 175
  pathogenesis 175
  treatment 176
Felix tube 63
Female anopheles mosquito 164
Fertility factor 13
Filamentous fungi 212
Filarial worms 207
Filtration 6
Fish tapeworm 184
Fitz-Hugh-Curtis syndrome 43, 99
Flocculation 24
Fluorescent treponemal antibody (FTA) 85
Frie's intradermal test 100
Fusobacterium 65

G

Gamma hemolysis 9
Gas gangrene 50
  clinical features 50
  lab diagnosis 50
  pathogenesis 50
  prophylaxis and treatment 51
Gastrodiscoides hominis 175
Gene transfer
  generalized 12
  lysogenic conversion 12
  mechanism 12f
  restricted 12
  transduction 12
  transformation 12
German measles 134
Giardia lamblia 153
  lab diagnosis 154
  life cycle 154
  morphology 153
  pathogenicity 154
  treatment 154
Gnathostoma spinigerum 211
Gonococcal bacteremia 43
Gonococci 44
Good pasteur's syndrome 31, 33
Gram staining 239
  procedure 239

H

Hacek group bacteria 69
Haemophilus ducreyi 69
  lab diagnosis 69
  treatment 69

Haemophilus influenzae 68
    lab diagnosis 68
    pathogenicity 68
Hand foot and mouth disease 139
Haptens 20
Hashimoto thyroiditis 33
HbCAg 129
HbEAg 129
HbSAg 128
Helicobacter pylori 92
    clinical features 92
    lab diagnosis 92
    mechanism of transmission 92
    pathogenicity 92
    treatment 92
Hemoflagellates 166
Hepatitis
    immunization 129
Hepatitis A 126
    clinical features 126
    pathogenesis 126
    prophylaxis 126
Hepatitis B 236
Hepatitis B virus 127
    antigenic diversity 127
    epidemiology 128
    lab diagnosis 128
    transmission 128
Hepatitis C virus 130
    clinical features 130
    lab diagnosis 130
    prophylaxis 130
    treatment 130
Hepatitis virus 126
Herpangina 139
Herpes simplex 109
    clinical features 109
        cutaneous 109
        encephalitis 110
        genital 110
        herpetic keratitis 109
        lab diagnosis 110
        mucosal 109
        visceral 110
    pathogenesis 109
Herpes viruses 108
    alpha 108
    beta 108
    gamma 109
Herpes zoster 112
    complications 112
HHV 3-varicella zoster virus 111
HHV 4-Epstien Barr virus 112
    causes 112
    pathogenicity 112

HHV 5-cytomegalovirus 113
    clinical features 113
    lab diagnosis 113
    prevention and treatment 113
HIB vaccine 237
Hide porter's disease 48
Histoplasmosis 224
Hookworm 196
Hot air oven 5
HSV-1 109
HSV-2 109
Human immunodeficiency virus 141
    antigen diversity 141
    clinical features 142
    group I 142
    group II 142
    group III 142
    group IV 142
    modes of transmission 145
    pathogenicity 141
    postexposure prophylaxis 145
Human trematodes 186
Hymenolepis nana 183, 195
Hypersensitivity 29
    delayed 29
    immediate 29
    type 1 29
        diagnosis 30
        effects 30
        mechanism 29
        prevention 30
    type 2 30
        mechanism 31
    type 3 31
        associated diseases 31
        effects 31
        mechanism 31
    type 4 32
    type 5 32
        mechanism 32

I

Idiopathic thrombocytopenic purpura 33
Immunity
    active 18
    adaptive 18
    artificial 19
    natural 19
    passive 19
    types 18
Immunodiffusion 24
Immunofluorescence 28, 28*f*
    direct 28
    indirect 28

Immunogenicity 20
Immunoglobulin 20
Immunoglobulin A 21
Immunoglobulin D 22
Immunoglobulin E 22
Immunoglobulin G 21
Immunoglobulin M 21
Immunological reaction 20
Immunology 18
Incineration 5
Indicator media 9
Infection 16
    method of transmission 16
    source of 16
Infectious diseases
    types 17
Influenza 114
    causes 114
    chemoprophylaxis 116
    clinical features 115
    immunoprophylaxis 116
    lab diagnosis 115
    pathogenicity 115
    types 115
        antigenic drift 115
        antigenic shift 115
Influenza virus 114
    morphology 114
Inspissation 5
Interferon 104
    biological effects 104
    clinical uses 104
    IFN-A 104
    IFN-B 104
    IFN-Γ 104
    types 104
Intestinal amebiasis 148
    pathogenesis 148
Intestinal flukes 175

J

Japanese encephalitis 122
    lab diagnosis 122
Jumping genes 15

K

Koch's postulates 1
Kyasanur forest disease 123
    clinical features 123
    lab diagnosis 123

L

Lancefield technique 24
Lansoprazole
    in *helicobacter pylori* 92

Larva migrans 186
Laryngoepiglottitis 68
Lecithinase effect 51
Legionella pneumophila 92, 235
    clinical features 93
    lab diagnosis 93
    pathogenicity 93
    treatment 93
Lepra reactions: 76
Lepromin test 77
    early reaction of fernandez 77
    late reaction of mitsuda 77
    uses of 77
Leprosy 76
    lab diagnosis 77
    madrid classification 76
    Ridley and Jopling classification 76
    treatment 77
    tuberculoid 76
Leptospira 85, 235
    lab diagnosis 86
    pathogenesis 85
    prophylaxis 87
    symptoms 86
    treatment 87
Leptospira icterohemorrhagiae 85
Leptospira interrogans 85
Liquid media 8
    disadvantages 8
    uses 8
Listeria monocytogenes 90
Live oral vaccine 238
Liver flukes 179
Loa loa 210
    life cycle 210
    pathogenicity and clinical features 211
    treatment 211
Loeffler's serum slope 70
Loeffler's syndrome 187
Long actin thyroid stimulator (LATS) 32
Lowenstein-Jensen medium 9
Lung flukes 176
Lyme disease 87
    epidemiology 87
    lab diagnosis 87
    pathogenesis 87
    treatment 87
Lymphatic filariasis 207

M

Malaria 163
    causative agents 163
    clinical features 164
    lab diagnosis 165
    pathogenesis 164

treatment 166
vector 164
Malassezia furfur 215
Malignant tertian malaria 164
Mantoux test 80
   interpretation 80
Mcconkey agar 9
Mcintosh and Fildes anaerobic jar 11
Mcintosh-fildes anaerobic jar 10
Measles 119
   clinical features 119
   lab diagnosis 119
   pathogenesis 119
   prophylaxis 120
Melioidosis 73
   lab diagnosis 73
   pathogenesis 73
   serology 73
   treatment 73
Membrane filter 6
Meningitis 68
Meningococcemia 42
Meningococci 44
Merozoite induced malaria 165
Metastatic amebiasis 149
Methicillin resistant Staphylococcus aureus 40
Microfilariae 210
MMR vaccine 236, 135
Moist heat 5
Monoclonal antibodies 23
   uses 23
Morbillivirus 119
Mucormycosis 228
Multiple myeloma 23
Mumps 117
   clinical features 118
   complications 118
   lab diagnosis 118
   pathogenesis 118
   prophylaxis 119
Mumps virus 117f
Myasthenia 33
Mycetism 231
Mycetoma 219
   diagnosis 219
   pathogenesis 219
   treatment 220
Mycobacterium tuberculosis 78
   antibiotic sensitivity testing 79
   culture 79
   decontamination 79
   microscopy 79
   mode of infection 78
   pathogenicity 78

Mycoplasma 88, 235
   morphology 88
Mycoses
   classification 214
Mycotic poisoning 231
Mycotoxicosis 231

N

Naegleria fowleri 150
   lab diagnosis 151
   life cycle 151
   morphology 150
   pathogenesis 151
   treatment 151
Nagler reaction 51
Necator americanus 198
Negri bodies 125
Neil mooser reaction 96
Neisseria 235
Neisseria gonorrhea 41, 42
   antigenic properties 42
   lab diagnosis 43
   pathogenicity 43
   penicillinase producing 44
   treatment 44
Neisseria meningitidis 41
   lab diagnosis 42
   pathogenesis 41
   prophylaxis 42
   treatment 42
Nematodes 186
New typhoid vaccine 238
Non gonococcal urethritis 44
   cause 44
Non-sporing anaerobes 65
   common diseases 65
   lab diagnosis 65
   treatment 65
Nontuberculous mycobacterium 81
   lab diagnosis 81
   mac complex 81
   runyoun classification 81
   skin pathogens 81
Nutrient agar 8
Nutrient broth 8

O

Occult filariasis 208
Oculomycosis 230
   pathogenesis and clinical features 230
   treatment 230
Oncogenesis 136
Oncogenic DNA viruses 136
Oncogenic RNA viruses 136

Oncogenic viruses 135
Ophthalmia neonatorum 43
OPV 236
Orthomyxoviridae 117
Orthomyxoviruses 114
Otomycosis 230
    causative agents 230

P

Pandemic 17
Papovaviruses 135
Paragonimus westermani 176
Parainfluenza virus 120
Paramyxoviridae 117
Parasites 146
    facultative 146
    free living 146
    obligate 146
Paratope 20
Passive agglutination test 25
Pencillin
    in streptococcus pneumoniae 37
Penicillin G
    in anthrax 49
    in streptoccocal infection 35
Penicilliosis 227
Peptococcus 65
Peptostreptococcus 65
Pernicious anemia 33
Picornaviruses 137
    classification 137
    lab diagnosis 138
Piedra 216
Pike's medium 35
Piperacillin
    Pseudomonas aeruginosa 73
Pityriasis versicolor 215
    clinical features 215
Plasmodium falciparum 163
Plasmodium malariae 164
Plasmodium ovale 164
Plasmodium vivax 163
Pneumococcal vaccine 237
Pneumocystis jirovecii 159
    clinical features 160
    life cycle 159f
    morphology 159
    pathogenesis 159
    treatment 160
Pneumonia 68
Poliovirus 137
    clinical features 138
    pathogenesis 137
Polyvalent polysaccharide vaccine 37
Post-tracheostomy pulmonary infections 72

Praziquantel 185
Precipitation 24
Precipitation reactions 24
    applications 24
    post zone phenomenon 24
    prozone phenomenon 24
    zone of equivalence 24
Prereduced anaerobic system (PRAS) 11
Primaquine 166
Prion disease 131
    animals 132
    human 132
    pathogenesis 131
    pathology 131
Progressive multifocal leukoencephalopathy 132
Prosodemic 17
Pseudomonas aeruginosa 72
    lab diagnosis 72
    pathogenicity 72
    treatment 73
Pseudophyllidea 183
Psittacosis 100
Pulmonary amebiasis 149
Pulse polio immunisation programme (PPI) 139
    objectives 139
Pyemia 17
Pyocyanin 72
Pyomelanin 72
Pyorubin 72
Pyoverdin 72

Q

Q fever 96
    lab diagnosis 97
    pathogenesis 96
Quantitative buffy coat (QBC) test 165
Quellung reaction 1

R

Rabies 237
    postexposure prophylaxis 237
Rabies virus 124
    antigenic properties 124
    host range 124
    lab diagnosis 125
    morphology 124
    pathogenesis 124
    prophylaxis 125
Radiation 6
    ionizing 6
    nonionizing 6
Recrudescent typhus 95
Reiter protein complement fixation 85
Reiter's syndrome 44, 99

Resistance transfer factor 14
Respiratory syncytial virus 120
    lab diagnosis 120
R factor 14
Rheumatoid arthritis 31, 33
Rhinosporidiosis 221
    diagnosis 222
    pathogenesis and clinical features 222
    treatment 222
Rickettsia prowazekii 94
Rickettsia typhi 94
Rickettsia 94
Rickettsiaceae 94
Rickettsial diseases 95
    lab diagnosis 95
    pathogenesis 95
    treatment 96
Rifampicin
    in Neisseria meningitidis 42
Robertson's cooked meat medium 11
Rotavirus 133
    clinical features 133
    lab diagnosis 133
    morphology 133
    pathogenesis 133
Rubella 134
    in pregnancy 134
    lab diagnosis 135
Rubella virus 134
    clinical features 134
    pathogenicity 134
    prophylaxis 135
Rubulavirus 117, 118

S

Salmonella 235
Satellitism 69
    prevention 69
    treatment 69
Scalded skin syndrome 38
Schistosomes 177
    hematobium 177
    japonicum 177
    mansoni 177
Scrub typhus 95
Seitz filter 6
Selective media 9
Septicemia 17
Serological reactions 24
Severe acute respiratory syndrome (SARS) 135
    clinical features 135
    prophylaxis 135
Sexduction 14f

Shigella 59
Shigella dysenteriae 59
    exotoxin 60
    invasive property 60
    pathogenicity 60
Simple media 8
SLE 31, 33
Slide coagulase test 40
Solid media 8
Spine like pseudopods 151
Spirochetes 82
Sporotrichosis 221
    causative agent 221
    pathogenesis and clinical features 221
    treatment 221
Standard test for syphilis 84
Staphylococcus 38
    bacteremia 38
    pathogenesis 38
    pyemia 38
    pyogenic infection 38
    septicemia 38
    toxin mediated disease 38
    toxins 39
        cytolytic 39
        enterotoxin 39
        epidermolytic 39
    treatment 40
    urinary tract infection 38
    virulence factors 38
Staphylococcus aureus 36, 235
Staphylococcus typhi 61
    antigenic structure 62
    lab diagnosis 62
    variations 62
Sterilization 4
Sterilizing agents 4
    chemical agents 4
        alcohols 7
        aldehydes 7
        antiseptics 7
        gaseous disinfectants 7
        phenols 7
        surface acting agents 7
    heat 4
    physical agents 4
        autoclave 5
        cold sterilization 7
        filtration 6
        radiation 6
Streptococcus MG test 89
Streptococcus pneumoniae 36, 235
    pathogenecity and clinical features 36
    prophylaxis 37

toxins and virulence factors 36
treatment 37
Streptococcus pyogenes 34, 235
    lab diagnosis 35, 37
    nonsuppurative 35
    pathogenicity 34
    prophylaxis 35
    respiratory infections 34
    skin and soft tissue infections 34
    structure 34, 36
    suppurative 34
    toxins 34
    treatment 35
Streptomycin
    in Brucella melitensis 75
Strongyloides stercoralis 200
    clinical features 201
    life cycle 201
STS *See* standard test for syphilis
Stuart's media 10
Subcutaneous mycoses 219
Swimming pool granuloma 81
Syphilis
    clinical features 83
    congenital 83
    lab diagnosis of 84
    latent 83
    primary 83
    secondary 83
    specific tests 85
    tertiary 83
    treatment 85

T

Tab vaccine 64
Taenia saginata 192, 195
    lab diagnosis 193
    life cycle 193
    morphology 192
    pathogenicity 193
    treatment 193
Taenia solium 194
    clinical features 195
    life cycle 194, 195
Tapeworms 183
Tetanus 53
    clinical features 53
    culture 53
    immunization 53
        active 53
        passive 53
    lab diagnosis 53
    pathogenesis 53

prophylaxis 53, 54
treatment 54
Thioglycolate broth 11
Tinea nigra 215
    diagonosis 215
Toxic shock syndrome 38, 39
    laboratory diagnosis 39
Toxin corregulated pilus (TCP) 45
Toxoplasma gondii 161
    life cycle of 162*f*
    prophylaxis 162
Trachoma 99
Transfer factor 13
Transport media 10
Transposition 15
Transposons 15
Traveller's diarrhea 58
Trematodes 174
Treponema 65, 82
Treponemaendemicum 82
Treponema pallidum 82
    antigenic structure 82
    mode of transmission 83
Treponema pallidum hemagglutination assay (TPHA) 85
Treponema pallidum immobilization 85
Trichinella spiralis 188
    clinical features 188
    life cycle 188
    morphology 188
    pathogenicity 188
    treatment 188
Trichomonas 155
    clinical features 156
    life cycle 155
    morphology 155
    pathogenesis 156
    treatment 156
Trichomonas vaginalis 44
Trichuris trichiura 198
    life cycle 199
    morphology 198
    treatment 200
Tropical pulmonary eosinophilia 209
Tropical splenomegaly syndrome 165
Trypanosoma brucei gambiense 166
Trypanosoma brucei rhodesiense 168
Trypanosoma cruzi 168
TT 236
Tube coagulase test 40
Tuberculin antigen 32
Tuberculosis 78
    extrapulmonary 79
    lab diagnosis 79
    MDR 80

    primary 78
    pulmonary 79
    secondary 78
    treatment 80
Tyndallization 5
Typhoid vaccine 238
Typhus fever 94
Tzanck smear 110

U

Ureaplasma urealyticum 89
Urinary tract infection 56
    culture 56
    lab diagnosis 57
    risk factors 56
    screening 56

V

Vancomycin
    in streptococcus pneumoniae 37
VDRL test 24
Venereal disease research laboratory (VDRL)
    test 84
Vibrio cholera 45
Viral hemagglutination 101
Virulence determinants 17
Viruses 101
    cell culture 102
    classification of 103
    cultivation of 102
        animal inoculation 102
        embryonated eggs 102
        tissue culture 102
    host interactions 103
    morphology 101
Visceral larva migrans 187
    clinical features 187
    diagnosis 187
    pathogenesis 187
    treatment 187

W

Weil felix reaction 96
West African trypanosomiasis 166
Widal test 63
    advantages 64
    interpretation of results 64
    procedure 64
Wuchereria bancrofti 207
    clinical features 208, 209
    life cycle 208

Y

Yeast 212
Yeast like 212
Yellow fever 122
    clinical features 122

Z

Ziehl-Neelsen staining 240
Zoophilic nematodes 186
Zygomycosis 228
    pathogenesis and clinical features 228
    treatment 229

EU GSPR Authorised Reprsentative
Logos Europe, 9 rue Nicolas Poussin
1700, La Rochelle, France
Phone: +33 (0) 6 67 93 73 78
E-mail: contact@logoseurope.eu

www.ingramcontent.com/pod-product-compliance
Ingram Content Group UK Ltd.
Pitfield, Milton Keynes, MK11 3LW, UK
UKHW051848210426

5322IPUK00024B/605